The Doctors' Plot of 1953

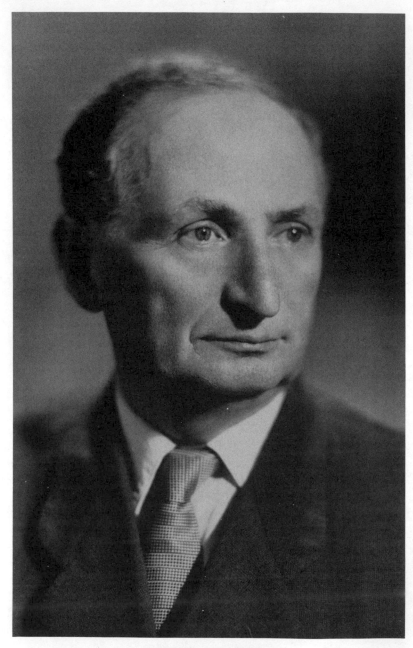

Yakov Rapoport, 1968

THE DOCTORS' PLOT
OF 1953

—

Yakov Rapoport

—

Harvard University Press
Cambridge, Massachusetts
1991

Original Russian-language edition published in Moscow, copyright © 1988
by Izdatelstvo KNIGA, who commissioned this English-language translation
by N. A. Perova and R. S. Bobrova

This book is printed on acid-free paper, and its binding materials have
been chosen for strength and durability.

LIBRARY OF CONGRESS CATALOGING-IN-PUBLICATION DATA

Rapoport, IA. L. (IAkov L'vovich), 1898–
[Na rubezhe dvukh ėpokh. English]
The doctors' plot of 1953 / Yakov Rapoport.
p.   cm.
Translation of: Na rubezhe dvukh ėpokh.
Includes index.
ISBN 0–674–21477–3
1. Rapoport, IA, L. (IAkov L'vovich).   2. Jews—Soviet Union—
Biography.   3. Political prisoners—Soviet Union—Biography.
Pathologists—Soviet Union—Biography.   5. Refuseniks—Biography.
6. Soviet Union—History—1925–1953—Biography.   I. Title.
DS135.R95R3713   1991
947'.00492402—dc20   90–4812
[B]   CIP

To my wife,
Sophia Rapoport

Preface

Those who are born in times of chaos
Cannot recall the paths they took.
We children of Russia's years of terror—
We have no power to forget.

ALTHOUGH THESE LINES of Alexander Blok refer to the fairly distant past, the early decades of this century, they are still relevant today. Moreover, they seem prophetic.

I entered life at the end of the nineteenth century and have lived to the end of the twentieth. There is little need to remind the reader what a tempestuous age this has been and what global changes have been wrought. Its dramatic events also found reflection in the microworld of Soviet medicine in which I spent the greater part of my life and to which I gave my mind and heart.

Let us return to the epigraph. One often hears today that many events of our grim past would be better forgotten (particularly from those who have a vested interest in such forgetting). "Why harp on tragedy?" these people ask. "Why mar the joyful present?" The great poet Blok maintained that the "children of Russia's years of terror" cannot forget. Can we who lived through the terror-filled years of midcentury forget them? Should we? This is not a question of coming to terms with our own feelings. It is a question of our duty to younger generations and to history.

It is our responsibility to reveal the whole truth of the life we lived, a truth that was suppressed for many years. A scientific approach to history requires more than documentary materials; eyewitness accounts, memoirs, and works of fiction are also of extreme importance. Such writings complement and illuminate documents and, as historical research testifies, often render inestimable assistance in reconstructing an epoch.

I wrote the first draft of this book almost in one sitting, relying principally on my memory, which continues to serve me faithfully in my advanced years. I did not then (in 1973) and do not now have access to any documents. Nor did I feel that I needed them: after all I am not, properly speaking, a historian. What I set out to do was to give an objective and full description, of necessity colored by certain natural emotions, of the events to which I was an eyewitness and of which I was a victim. I have drawn on very few written sources to fill out my story.

I was in a hurry to write, for the years were pressing in and I was afraid I might not be granted time to finish. To be sure, with more time and greater access to information, the interpretation of the facts contained in this book might undergo changes: thinking never remains stationary. And possibly, if I were describing certain events today and not some fifteen years ago, the perspective might be different. But this task I leave for the reader, and I see no point in altering the texture of my book.

The Doctors' Plot was the culmination of thirty years of Stalin's rule, a regime of lawlessness and terror, and it marked the end of that era. I regard it as a debt of gratitude to remind readers of the energetic actions the country's new leadership took in the first days after Stalin's death, quashing the doctors' case and taking measures to restore justice and legality. I want particularly to mention the courageous stand taken by Nikita Khrushchev.

My friends and students urged me to leave a literary record of my life experience and particularly of the Doctors' Plot. It was my civic duty, they argued. I heeded their arguments because they coincided with my own desires and intentions. So you may take this book as a testament to my life and times.

Y. L. R.
Moscow, 1988

Contents

The Doctors' Plot of 1953

Prologue: Memory Is Medicine

Natalya Rapoport

THESE EVENTS of my childhood have lain hidden in the depths of my soul for all these years, but I have never ceased to feel their scorching pain.

At the age of fourteen I was an unbelievably naive and cheerful child. Even after the official broadcast, on January 13, 1953, announcing the discovery of a "criminal group of killer doctors" and "murderers in white coats," I did not anticipate any personal misfortune, although many family friends were among the accused.

Some two weeks later, on the night of February 2, my father was arrested. Catastrophe swooped down on me like a tornado. Thirty-seven years have passed since that time, and life has granted me many happy personal encounters. But still I try to fit all new friends and acquaintances into those years: how would they have behaved?

I can't guarantee the documentary accuracy of my story: I describe these events as preserved in the admittedly turbulent memory of a child. But nothing is fabricated; I simply present one small segment of my generation's history.

Fortunate people pass smoothly from childhood to adulthood, managing along the way to delight in each changing stage. But I was catapulted out of my childhood. The catapult was triggered by our concierge, Lucia, when the doorbell exploded into the late-night silence of our apartment. As often happened in those days, my parents were out. The sudden ring at such an hour startled me.

"Who's there?"

"Natasha, open up! There's something wrong with your heating system," answered the door with Lucia's voice.

I was surprised—nothing was wrong with our heating system.

"Natasha, open the door immediately! Your radiator is leaking, the neighbors below are complaining," Lucia insisted.

I opened the door. Standing there was a gang of thugs, so many that our stairwell could hardly hold them. One or two were disguised in military uniform; the others, in civilian clothes, all looked remarkably alike.

Instantly our apartment was inundated. Crowding me against the wall, they poured into the flat in a violent stream. At the end of our hallway, this stream divided into separate streamlets, flowing into my father's study, the dining room, the kitchen, the washroom and even the toilet. One of the "officers" sat in the dining room and presided like a host. All the others reported to him: "Bookcases—six; wardrobes—three; cupboards—five; writing desks . . . beds . . ."

I became less anxious: "They've come to steal the furniture, and they're not going to kill me after all," I reassured myself. I didn't care about the furniture; to be honest, I had always resented the way my father complained about glue on the piano keys, paint on the sofa, or scratches on the table. "Maybe everything will come out all right," I thought, hiding behind the sofa in my room. The only thing I prayed they wouldn't take was the piano. It was an heirloom, recovered from our bombed-out house on Starokonyushenye Lane during the war. I was only three at the time. My parents had returned from the country to find our house in ruins, with the piano suspended from a bare girder like a spirit. It could never be tuned again, but everyone liked and admired it. I felt sorry for the piano.

Strangely, the thieves were in no hurry at all. They examined the apartment meticulously, each corner, every inch, and I started to worry again. Any minute now my parents could return, and I was terrified to think what would happen then. My father is a proud, hot-tempered man who wouldn't care about the odds against him. He would protest violently, and the bastards would kill all of us. My teeth clattered loudly, uncontrollably.

Suddenly the telephone rang, making my heart almost stop, and one of the thieves grabbed me: "Hurry up, answer the phone, but say nothing about us being here—understand?" My legs wouldn't obey me. The man dragged me across the floor, almost carrying me the last few feet. He lifted the receiver, thrust it against my ear, and hissed, "Answer!"

Only my parents would call at one in the morning. My throat contracted in a spasm and I couldn't say a word. "Natalochka— you're not asleep yet?" asked my mother anxiously. "We'll be home soon."

It was absolutely terrifying, and too much for me. I fainted.

Both my parents were doctors. My father was a world-famous pathologist, with a reputation not only for his professional skills but also for his wit. Perhaps he tried to compensate for the grimness of his profession with jokes. These were known throughout Moscow, and I committed them to memory for the time when I would be old enough to understand them.

One time I remember Papa telling his friends about the dilemma of the bureaucrats who were being pressured to fire the director of the Second Medical Institute, Abram Borisovich Topchan. Everybody liked Topchan, both professors and students. For a long time the bureaucrats couldn't find an appropriate excuse. At last, without concocting anything, they simply announced, "Topchan, Abram Borisovich, is dismissed."

"What idiots," my father scoffed. "They should have phrased it 'Topchan, being Abraham Borisovich [a distinctly Jewish name], is dismissed.'"

All Papa's friends laughed, but I felt somehow that it was not happy laughter. This was 1948.

Moscow biologists were also highly amused when my father

proposed marriage to the venerable septuagenarian, the pseudo-scientist Lepeshinskaya, who received a Stalin Prize for her "outstanding discovery of the vital substance." (I studied this at school.)

"Olga Borisovna," my father said, "you are now the most desirable girl in Moscow. Would you marry me and we'll make children from the vital substance?" Malicious tongues wagged: they said she was pleased with the first part of the proposal, but not with the second.

So my father used to make jokes at a time when biologists and doctors no longer had any reason to laugh.

My mother was a physiologist. Most of her life she worked with Lina Stern, the preeminent woman academician in the Soviet Union. Lina came from a rich family in western Europe, studied in Geneva, and left everything to come to the Soviet Union in the mid-1920s, captivated by the idea of participating in the most progressive society on earth. With typical humor, she once told me why she had become a scientist. Lina had a beautiful younger sister. Their father arranged a debutante ball for Lina, where her sister was a glittering success: all the most eligible young men invited her to dance, forgetting all about the other sister. "And it was at that moment," Lina said, "that I realized my destiny was science." She was devoted to this cause for all the ninety years of her remarkable life, and she died a virgin.

Lina was talented, brilliant, and domineering, with a sharp tongue. Back then I was afraid of her. She demanded that her colleagues match her own total dedication to work, but others had husbands, wives, children. Returning from wartime Siberian evacuation, my mother had trouble placing me in a kindergarten, so she took me along with her to the institute, deadly afraid that Lina would discover me. I spent part of my childhood in a laboratory cupboard that was specially emptied for me to hide in whenever Lina entered. (Was it then that my interest in natural science was born?) Sitting there in shadowed silence, I listened to the laboratory sounds: the zzzhhh of an

4

instrument recording the rhythms of frogs' heartbeats and muscular contractions; the clicking of thermostats; the shrill voice of Lina, swearing at her colleagues.

Once my mother could no longer bear it and said, "Lina Solomonova, please don't swear at the senior scientists in the presence of juniors—it undermines our authority. Take us to your office and curse there as much as you like."

"But by the time I reach my office all my anger will have evaporated," replied Lina. (Her office was only two steps away, but that's what Lina was like.)

My mother literally divided herself between work and family, which she loved to the point of complete self-denial. Unfortunately I was prone to illness, the legacy of my cold and hungry childhood in wartime Siberia.

"Sophia Yakovlevna, why does Natashenka get sick so often?" Lina used to ask accusingly. "Perhaps you don't pay enough attention to her."

Enough attention? Oh, no! Lina and the institute took at least three quarters of Mama's time and always tried to take the rest. A vital detail: Lina and I were born on the same date, August 26, separated by sixty years. You can be sure, my mother always had to leave my birthday parties for Lina's: from my celebration, which my friends and I prepared all summer, with games, songs, and performances in which I was the star, to the dull old people whose life was almost behind them.

I was about ten years old when Lina suddenly disappeared from our lives. Vanished totally. My parents answered my questions in a very evasive way, and I didn't persist. Without Lina, my life became much better. Now my mother belonged to me completely; there was even a period of time when she didn't go to work. Of course I saw that my parents were terribly dispirited by Lina's disappearance, but at the bottom of my heart, secretly and shamefully, I relished the new situation. Now when I became ill, my mother was at my bedside; she read aloud to me from wonderful books and even played games with me. It was a joy to be sick!

5

When this joy lasted too long, Dr. Miron Vovsi was called. He looked at me with his kind, radiant eyes, examined me, touched the swollen joints, and reproached me: "I see by your eyes that you were running around again in the damp without buttoning up your coat, without a scarf! No? Why, I know you were! Wait a little, just a few years, you'll grow up, everything will pass away and then all the puddles will be yours!"

How nice! Just a few years. But at that time, a few years were a major portion of my life, from which Dr. Vovsi was blithely subtracting the best part. For example, he had me excused from physical fitness at school. While my whole class was excitedly chasing a ball down the hall, I had to sit on a bench by the window, completely humiliated.

Nevertheless, despite my frequent illnesses, I was remarkably well off during those years. Greedily I devoured the wisdom of the natural and exact sciences. Burning with impatience, I would race through my textbooks, faster, faster, what's next? With delight I would solve hard problems. In general, I lived as if surrounded by a rose-colored screen, basking in the warm rays of general approval. But outside my protective screen, some unimaginable horrors were occurring. One after another my parents' friends disappeared, and even in their own home my parents spoke their friends' names only in whispers. Yet I remained totally oblivious of the incomprehensible shape of the times. Other breezes were carrying me, only occasionally splashing me with their icy spray. One event in particular is etched in my memory.

In my childhood I used to compose verses. I was sure they were very good verses—they were even read at school ceremonies. Sometimes the author herself recited them; sometimes, if they were long, they were divided by sections among my schoolmates, and there were times when the whole class recited them in chorus:

> Among the trees
> The twittering birds

Gently are a-callin'
And with one voice
They all sing out
The name of Comrade Stalin.

I studied in Demonstration School No. 29. During recess the director, a horrible old hag called Martyanova, stood in the middle of the recreation hall, all in black, and the schoolgirls walked in sedate pairs along the perimeter around her. Though I was a good student and well behaved, I was terribly afraid of Martyanova. The old woman had a collection of important titles. Delegations often visited to see how happily Moscow schoolgirls lived and how diligently they studied. It was from our school that Young Pioneers were chosen to lead May 1st parades: running ahead of the columns of marchers to Lenin's tomb to present flowers to members of the government and to Comrade Stalin himself. Such an event excited my patriotic soul, and as a result the following lines were born:

Take courage, comrades—we're the best!
Stand up and let's away.
For this fine group of Pioneers
Will lead the march today!

Perhaps for this masterpiece, for past merits, for exemplary behavior, or maybe to demonstrate the victory of Lenin's nationality policy, I was to be included in that column of Pioneers. Even in my most fantastic dreams I couldn't imagine such joy—to stand on the Mausoleum right next to Comrade Stalin. My triumph was boundless! I boasted incessantly: to my neighborhood friends, relatives, and the not-yet arrested friends of my parents. Everyone, just everyone, had to witness my triumph.

But then the inconceivable happened. On the very eve of the celebration, only one step away from unutterable happiness and glory, my father with the sharp eye of a pathologist discovered inflamed tonsils in my throat (but I *always* had inflamed tonsils!). He pronounced me sick, sent me to bed, and wouldn't let me out. This was unheard of! Hadn't Papa forced me to go to school before, when I wanted to stay at home to read an interesting book and faked a sore throat? I almost drowned my parents in tears, but Papa, with whom one could generally come to terms, this time was adamant. Thus were my great dreams shattered, leaving an ugly scar of resentment toward my parents in my child's soul.

The years passed, and although the youngest in my class, I was the first to be accepted into the Komsomol. Exulting, I demanded that my parents organize a great celebration commensurate with my glorious success. But just outside my window it was November 1952, and with dizzying speed the guest chairs around my parents' hospitable table were emptying. The remaining friends came to us unrecognizable: nervous, distressed, unable to smile. My own parents had long since begun disappearing for hours at a time in the evenings. (I found out much later that they were expecting arrest any day and had been distributing to their few, still unimprisoned friends small sums of money and some of my warm clothing—for the north—so that, given the chance, someone could send me to my mother's camp.)

January 13, 1953. Oblivious, I am listening to the radio for the fifth time that day. I am accustomed to trusting it completely. Suddenly my brain refuses to comprehend what I hear. It just cannot be, it simply cannot be! Dr. Vovsi, Miron Semyonovich Vovsi, whose gentle hands and radiant eyes had always been there throughout my childhood and my illnesses. And other doctors too. I hadn't slighted any of them, falling ill equally for each according to his speciality. And now all of them, who had just recently been joking, laughing, hugging me in our warm and happy home, turned out to be killers, monster-freaks of the human race, evildoers dressed in white coats, with but a single goal—to murder the devoted leaders of the Communist Party and the government.

"It can't be!" I burst out, looking in shock at my shaken

parents. "Tell them it's a lie! Why are you standing there? Run and tell them!"

"Yes, it's a mistake," my grim-faced mother said in an unfamiliar, choked voice, carefully choosing her words. "It's a horrible mistake, and it will of course be cleared up soon. But don't tell anyone, understand, not anyone, that you don't believe this. You could bring a lot of harm to your father and me, and you"—here followed a terrifying threat—"you will be expelled from the Komsomol! Don't speak to anybody about this."

It was easy to say "don't speak about it," but everywhere—in school, around the neighborhood, on the buses and trolley cars, in the shops— there was just one conversation: the bloody crimes of the uncovered traitors. I tried to be patient, silent, but little by little I was going out of my mind. Where is the truth? Where is the lie? Where is north? Where is south? The ground gave way under my feet, and I was at a loss.

People cursed the bloody killers and everyone of the same "nationality." How they thirsted for revenge! The mass media whipped up these emotions, and people refused to be treated by Jewish doctors. The air reeked of pogrom. There were rumors that, for the sake of "protecting" the others—the innocent Jews—from all this mass hatred, camps were being set up for them in Siberia. All of them would be sent there very soon.

The question of how to execute the criminals was widely discussed. Informed circles in my class contended that they would be hanged in Red Square. Many worried about whether the execution would be open to the public or only to those with special permission. Some figured it would only be for those with permission, since otherwise the overcurious mob would stampede and destroy Lenin's tomb. Someone consoled the disappointed: "Don't worry; surely they'll film it." And only I dreamed of Vovsi on the gallows and woke up screaming.

During all this, not even for a second, not for a flashing thought, did I dream that this could happen to my father.

"Rapaport, to the blackboard!"

We couldn't stand our stupid, short-legged, malicious history teacher. Grating, grinding, she pulled an old ship along the dried-up river bed of her barren historical materialism. To listen to her, all human history was reduced to a sequence of changes from one social or economic structure to another, brought on by the contradictions between productive forces and productive relations. With the ruthlessness of a vivisectionist she dissected the living, pulsating flesh of history, forcing us to examine the cadaver. But today I was very happy that she had called on me. I liked the subject, the U.S. Constitution. I had even read something extra for the day's lesson and had run to my "Aunt" Julia for additional information.

Julia and Shabsai Moshkovsky were close family friends. We lived in the same apartment building, constructed by the medical cooperative MEDIK. We had moved there in 1951. All of the tenants were medical doctors with their families. Shabsai, for instance, was a corresponding member of the Academy of Medical Sciences. His wife, Aunt Julia, was a historian and specialist in medieval Germany. She graduated from Freiburg University and could speak about historical figures as if she were personally acquainted with them and historical events as if they had happened before her very eyes. I loved her stories. We were very close, and I shared confidences with her that even my parents never knew. This time Aunt Julia had told me the fascinating story of young America. And now in class I retold her tale with great pleasure. My classmates were all ears.

The history teacher gave me a C. The mark caused a sensation: for me, even a B was an event. I was stunned and my classmates were indignant. "What? She didn't answer correctly? What did she say wrong?"

"No, she answered correctly," the history teacher replied defensively. "But in what tone? With what intonation?" Suddenly she screeched mockingly, "Ah, what a wonderful country America is! I have an aunt in America! I will leave for America tomorrow!" Well, that was really too much. I quickly gathered my things and stormed out of the room, slamming the door behind me: "That's it! To hell with it! I'll never go to school again!"

My parents were very upset. Incredibly they were upset over such nonsense, when any moment could bring real disaster to them. Despite that looming danger, they went to the school director. In this, my new school, the director was a mathematician—as dry and strict as her discipline. Many years passed before I realized what a feat this woman accomplished. Unbelievably, she forced the history teacher to apologize publicly.

This happened at our next history lesson. The director accompanied the history teacher into the classroom and sat in the last row. Looking sideways slightly toward a portrait of Stalin on the wall, her eyes empty of expression, the teacher muttered limply, "I have reconsidered Rapoport's report in the previous class. Perhaps there was no groveling to America in her answer. But she didn't emphasize that since the time the constitution was ratified, many things have changed in America and that today there are no traces of the freedoms proclaimed in the constitution. Nevertheless, I have decided to change Rapoport's grade to a B. Give me the grade book."

Taken aback by this unexpected turn of events, I handed her my grade book. This class took place two days after the visit of our nighttime visitors, but the history teacher did not know she had apologized not to the Komsomol member and exemplary student Natasha Rapoport, but to the daughter of "a murderer, a member of an anti-Soviet terrorist organization." Such are the paradoxes of history.

. . . I had fainted so deeply that I didn't hear my parents return or my father being taken away. I regained consciousness much later, still in complete ignorance. Mama was kneeling next to me. A strange male voice asked:

"Is this your daughter?"

"Yes."

"Yours and the arrestee's?"

The arrestee? A powerful wave seized me, whirled me around, thrashing me, breaking my bones, and bearing me away forever from my rosy world, my happy childhood. I regained consciousness the second time as the daughter of a killer doctor.

In our apartment, the search continued. For these professionals the job is routine, boring, almost automatic. Every book, page by page. Every pillow, every drawer. Here they find a letter from my friend Jan, whom I befriended in Estonia last summer. They look it over, ask if I have more, take everything away. How could I have known that Jan's father was an imprisoned Estonian priest, an important leader of the Estonian church, and that my friendship with Jan would be one of the links in the chain of my father's criminal actions?

Boring, boring—now they've found several books by Freud. They leaf through them muttering, add them to the evidence. Now they've picked up a Finnish knife, a war trophy my father used for boating. Suddenly, a sensation! In the medicine cabinet, among other harmless ampules, they find one with a skull and crossbones and the inscription "Poison." Here it is at last— the necessary, irrefutable evidence. Everybody looks at the discoverer with respect and envy.

"And how many is it possible to put to sleep with one such ampule?" asks the lieutenant, the only one in military uniform at the search.

"It is not possible to kill *anybody* with this ampule," my mother tries to explain. "This is medicine, atropine, a remedy for heart disease. My husband had a heart attack, and we keep medicines at home to be on the safe side."

"Oh yes, I understand, of course, what you keep it for," says the lieutenant venomously. "I understand what kind of heart medicine you have here. Just how many hearts were stopped with this medicine?" He is happy.

All my mother's attempts to explain are in vain. They call somebody by telephone, informing them of the find. (It is late at night, but *there* they never sleep.) They wrap the ampule carefully in cotton wool, seal it into a small box and insert that into yet another box, which is also sealed. They draw up a document stating that poison was found in the arrestee's apartment and demand that my mother sign it. She categorically refuses. They urge, then threaten her. If she doesn't sign, she will have to go with them. For a long time? Forever? I am in despair. But Mama doesn't sign.

The excited mood of our visitors associated with finding the ampule soon evaporates. There has been an accident: one man has cut his finger on a razor blade, and there's a drop of blood. This unlucky fellow has cut his finger in the home of a killer doctor: his days are numbered. He is sitting in a chair, paler than the walls, his wounded hand extended. His comrades circle around him and worriedly discuss the situation. What to do? Can he be saved?

Mama proposes an inventive solution. She brings the distraught man iodine. The tension now hits its apogee: should the iodine be applied or not? One volunteer with courage born of despair puts a drop of iodine on his nail. One after another, each man sniffs it. It is decided not to take the risk. They phone somewhere for a car and the suffering one is taken away—most likely to a special clinic where his scratch will be treated by a trusted, dependable *Russian* surgeon.

The search is over. They have sealed the apartment and have left us my room, the hallway, kitchen, washroom, and toilet. As they had warned, Mama was taken away. Neither she nor I knew if we would see one another again.

But Mama did return, after twenty-four hours. It turned out that she was just taken to our dacha, which they also searched down to the last speck of dust. Mama later told me that upon her return she had found me in the same chair in the hall, just as she had left me. It seemed to her that I hadn't budged. I myself don't remember anything about those twenty-four hours except the heartbreaking howling of our dog Topsy. Most probably we were a duet.

With Mama, my life returned.

I was morbidly attached to my mother. In my childhood, when she would travel somewhere with Papa, I would simply fall ill, stop eating, vomit, and, it seemed to me, die until she returned. I would count the days, the hours, the minutes. I was prepared to do anything for my mother. Mama was always delighted with my successes, which, for a long time after her death, simply lost all meaning for me. During those days it was very important to my mother that my life not be disrupted by my father's arrest and that I continue going to school. So I went. But from that moment on, two fears took over my life, two fears that merged into one uninterrupted horror: the daytime fear that my classmates would uncover my disgrace; and the nighttime fear that my mother would be taken away.

The nighttime fear began at eleven and lasted until five in the morning. For some reason, I was convinced that she couldn't be arrested earlier or later. My fear was so strong that during those hours I trembled all over as if in a fit; I even slept in the hall on a cot rather than in my room, listening tensely the whole night to sounds and rustlings on the staircase; the slamming of the elevator door on the nearby floors made me cry out in terror.

The daytime fear held me in its grip during school hours, turning me into a small compressed spring. Only three girls in my class knew my secret, three girls who lived in my apartment building. Their parents sternly forbade them to breathe a word, even to their closest friends, probably thinking that tomorrow any of them might share the same fate. And the girls were silent, although it's easy to imagine how difficult it was to keep such a sensational secret. The secret, desperate to come out, burned the ends of their tongues.

I used all my strength to appear my usual cheerful self. But then one of the three girls broke down. During recess she took me aside: "You think we're keeping quiet so you can act as if you're a full and equal member of our group?" The months of tension exploded in a resounding slap that I planted on the face of my offender. In a flash the class closed in a circle around us: "What's happened?"

The advocate of the pure society looked at me with a mixture of astonishment and hate, and I, on the verge of fainting, hardly able to stand on trembling legs, was overpowered at the awful truth swelling up in her mouth, seeping through her teeth, and now here, at this very moment, about to burst from her lips . . . The bell rang! It released me from paralysis: I flew to class, feverishly gathered my things, and left school—perhaps forever.

How did we live? My mother was fired the morning after my father's arrest. All the money in the house as well as our bonds and savings passbook were taken during the search. There was, I believe, some method in this. They wanted to see who would come to our aid and, following this thread, could haul in the whole evil chain to the very last link. People understood this and were afraid. Encountering me in the street, neighbors averted their eyes, tried to slip by; they didn't recognize me. But not everyone. I will never forget our neighbors, Vladimir Nikolaevich and Nina Petrovna Beklemishev, from the old Russian intelligentsia. Vladimir was a tall, handsome man with a pointed beard, an academician who looked as if he had stepped out of the portraits of the great nineteenth-century scientists, aristocrats of the spirit. Whenever he met Mama in the street, he didn't simply greet her, he deeply bowed to her, displaying to others a conspicuous example of courage and nobility.

His wife Nina bravely came to our apartment right after Papa's arrest and offered us money. My mother didn't accept it—there was no way she could ever pay it back—but Nina would not leave until she received Mama's solemn promise to turn to her for help the moment she needed it, day or night.

Once I met Aunt Julia in the street, and she took me to her apartment. She fed me, questioned me about everything, gave me extra food for Mama, and quickly sent me on my way. God forbid that Shabsai should return from work and catch us—he would die of fear. Shabsai was a kind, interesting, and absolutely decent person who adored children and was adored by them in turn. I myself loved him dearly, although with a tinge of indulgence, finding him peculiar in many ways. Instead of tea, he drank only hot water of a most peculiar color, fastidiously washed his hands, ate only the freshest food, never allowed alcohol to touch his lips, and was in general extraordinarily circumspect.

In contrast, Aunt Julia enjoyed one or two glasses of wine at celebrations. Once her son, in first grade, wrote in response to a school survey about the drinking habits of his parents: "Father—sober. Mother—drinker." A worried teacher then came to their house and was most surprised when the door was opened by an extremely charming woman with a slender intelligent face; and on the walls she saw original paintings by famous artists with accompanying dedications. For a long time afterward, Aunt Julia was the butt of many jokes: "Julenka, don't drink so much, you remember what happened the last time!" Now, in comparison with the circumspection of Shabsai, Aunt Julia's taking me to their home smacked of heroism and I admired her for it.

Natashka Tomilina, a girl from our apartment building who was in my grade at school, would drop by. Before she had visited only rarely, now almost every day. She would take out the sandwich and apple from her school case: "Listen, eat up, huh? If my mother finds out I didn't eat lunch at school, she'll kill me." Not once did she glance at the sealed doors or ask why I sat on a cot in the hallway—just a normal thing, after all, a person living in a hallway on a cot. Natashka took out her textbooks: "Listen, help me with these physics problems. Look at the stupid stuff we studied today. Look."

To this day, Natashka claims that she did this without an ulterior motive: what kind of fool would rack her brains to solve those silly problems when there was a simpler, more elegant, and reliable way—just have me do it. She is most likely lying. She herself was an excellent student and could easily solve those "silly problems." But in any case, thanks to Natashka, I stayed abreast of school news, gossip, and the curriculum. When I returned to school I wasn't behind at all.

The classics also helped us to get through. There was a bookcase in the hall with the collected works of Tolstoy, Pushkin, Hugo. Mama took them to the bookstores, returning with bread, milk, and kasha. We survived. But the classics left our house in suspicious-looking, bulky sacks, and someone informed on us: Mama was selling things from behind the sealed doors. Again a search.

This time I almost died with fear. I thought they had come for Mama. They broke the intact seals, immediately saw that the accusation was false, but were obliged to verify everything from the beginning, according to the list. I took a fit, kicked and screamed. But they didn't take Mama. They sealed everything up again and left.

And there was one family who helped us unfailingly throughout.

My mother had shared the same desk with Raya Guber in high school. The friendship that developed lasted their entire lives; they were closer than sisters. When I was born, my mother fell ill with typhus, and Aunt Raya breast-fed me along with her own Marishka, who had been born two months earlier. They also had a son, Shurik, a year older.

"You were nursed at the breast of my own wife!" Andrey Alexandrovich Guber used to reproach me, with the clear implication that any person fed at *such* a breast should not have any shortcomings. The Gubers were my second family.

What an attractive couple! Aunt Raya—diminutive, graceful, joyous; Andrey—tall, elegant, gray-eyed, inventor and soul of our childhood games: lapta, lotto, catch, he played them all enthusiastically. Andrey was descended from Russified Germans, his ancestors having come to Russia during the reign of Peter the Great. He was an art critic, a professor at Moscow University, a specialist in Renaissance art, and head curator of the Pushkin Museum of Fine Art. He was a wonderful raconteur with whom my father composed extraordinary duets of storytelling; with those cadences we grew up.

17

The museum at that time was a second home for us. All the museum babushki knew us, as we hurried there to listen to lectures and flitted around the halls. Sometimes Andrey would take us down to the storage rooms to play.

Despite Andrey's high position, the Gubers had a very difficult life. They lived in a huge communal building, in a small room divided like a railroad car into compartments. That resemblance was underscored by the sleeping arrangements in which Shurik slept above Marishka in a bunk bed—there was simply not enough room for two regular beds. Books took up most of the available space. Friends would insist that Andrey obtain a better apartment, but he was consistently foiled: he lacked the necessary skill in battling or bribing bureaucrats. Finally, the opportunity came to buy a small cooperative apartment. But the move was his undoing. In sorting and packing his books, he overworked himself and had a heart attack. They could not save him.

The museum bid him farewell in the Italian courtyard. A small orchestra played light music, Tyutchev and Pushkin were read, and there was no sense that this was a funeral. It seemed that Andrey was still here. Michelangelo's David, the frescos on the walls, and the chimeras on the vaulted ceilings above us joined in our farewell. People spoke movingly of a man who would remain living forever among the treasures he had so lovingly preserved.

And I recalled how, in those terrible days, Andrey had sent Marishka to our house and how he had ordered me to come to their home every day for dinner. My daily visits were a tremendous risk for the Gubers, the more so since they lived in a communal building where any tenant could inform on them. But the Gubers were beyond fear. They took me in each day, fed me, gave me food for Mama and packages for Papa. These trips I will never forget.

In our stairwell, in the street, in the courtyard, there were always MGB agents waiting to follow us. I could easily pick them out of a crowd—it wasn't at all difficult. Mama taught me how to lose them. I would go into the subway, get into a car, and stand close to a door. As the doors were closing, I quickly jumped out, hopped on a train coming in the opposite direction, and rode for two or three stations. On my way from Sokol to the center of town, I would repeat the operation several times. I had to be absolutely sure I had lost them; otherwise I was supposed to return home. I don't remember ever failing to lose my bloodhounds. But to go out into the street was torture for another reason.

There were barrack-like tenements in our courtyard. After Papa's arrest and even before morning broke, the inhabitants of the barracks had already informed everyone around that my father had taken pus from cancerous corpses and rubbed it into the skin of healthy people. The young boys from the barracks enthusiastically took it upon themselves to avenge my father's monstrous crimes, hurling at me everything they could get their hands on—rotten vegetables, dead mice and rats, and sometimes even cobblestones. No matter how humiliating it was, I had to turn tail and run; if I wasn't fast enough, I would get a beating.

One day in February 1953 my mother returned home looking like death; they hadn't accepted a package for my imprisoned father. "Don't bring any more, they are no longer necessary," said the MGB man on duty, looking at some list. He refused to answer Mama's questions. There could be only one explanation: Papa was no longer alive.

The days dragged on—bleak, empty, dark.

March 4, 1953. Stalin is ill. Mama can't tear herself away from the radio—tensely, eagerly she listens. Cheyne-Stokes breathing, the end is near. Mama is silent, waiting.

March 5, 1953. It is finished! For the first time, some kind of faint, uncertain light penetrates the black night of my mother's eyes. If only Papa were alive—so much could change now!

The 8th or 9th of March. A phone call. A male voice spoke: "I am calling at the request of the professor. The professor asked me to tell you that he is healthy, feels fine, and is concerned about his family. What should I say to the professor?" Do you understand? Not the murderer, not the monster, not the scum of the earth—but the *professor*. He is alive!

"We are fine," my mother almost screams. "Tell him we are fine, we are healthy, we are—happy!" (This was hardly an appropriate word to end a speech in those days of national mourning.)

He is alive! With my earth-shaking news I fly to the Gubers. They embrace me, cry with me, and Aunt Raya runs to the kitchen for cake. "For the wake," she awkwardly lies to the shocked neighbors. "We want to remember Joseph Vissarionovich in the Russian tradition!" I fly back home with cake and treats for the great celebration.

He is still in the Hall of Columns. Yet even his corpse thirsts for new victims, as hundreds of onlookers—mourners and the merely curious—are trampled to death in the crowd coming to view the body. But at our home there is a celebration. For the first time in my life I feel my alienation piercingly and acutely, and I am conscious of it not as a child but as a grown-up. It is the beginning of my adulthood.

Now my mother and I live on hope. Mama again sends off packages. It turns out that Papa had been in special confinement and, among other things, had not been allowed to receive packages. We learn later that he refused to sign the false accusations against either himself or others, and they transferred him to a special prison to persuade him otherwise. But even then he didn't sign.

Days and weeks pass. No news, no news.

Then late on the night of April 3rd, our dog Topsy suddenly goes wild. She starts running up and down the hallway, banging up against the sealed door of the dining room, then against the door to the stairwell, clearing my cot with a single bound. I'm in a panic: they're coming to arrest Mama!

The telephone rings. My father's voice: "My darlings, it's me! I'll be home in an instant. I'm calling from the telephone booth downstairs. I didn't want you to faint at my sudden appearance."

Topsy sits frozen at the door; only her tail wags like a pendulum back and forth, back and forth. She is whining impatiently. After a minute, the doorbell rings. Papa! With him is a MGB colonel and the same lieutenant who had taken him away—now he carries Papa's little suitcase. Topsy is the first to greet him: with a record leap from the floor she is at his neck, licking his lips, nose, eyes. Next it is my mother's turn, then mine. We laugh and cry, all at once.

The colonel says, "We return the professor to you." While the lieutenant removes the seals from the doors, the colonel telephones somewhere: "Comrade General, the professor has been delivered. There is much joy, many tears."

The solemn black suit pinned with the Order of Lenin droops on my father as though on a hanger. The Order of Lenin, which he received for wartime service, now dazzles our eyes. At home! Alive, and with a certificate of full rehabilitation! Here it is—the certificate—we look at it, hold it up to the light, but can't read; at this moment we're having trouble comprehending anything.

The colonel says that later this afternoon all our confiscated things will be returned; he wishes us luck and they leave. The three of us are alone. Papa, Mama, and I. Papa talks, Mama listens. I don't hear a thing—I just look at Papa.

Six o'clock in the morning. The radio announces to all the world the end of the killer-doctor affair and the full rehabilitation of all the accused. The doorbell rings: our neighbors, the Beklemishevs, and behind them the Kaplans. They hadn't slept all night, hearing the noise and thinking they had come to take my mother. But then—the radio.

From that moment the door of our apartment never closes; within a few hours the entire building has come to visit. Flowers, flowers. Quite unexpectedly, my entire school class shows up; now there is no need to keep secrets, and those girls "in the know" are rewarded for their months of silence by their pride in having kept it. Everyone comes, even my tormenter, with a flower in hand! One by one, each gives a flower to Papa. I am crying. (Even now I am crying as I write these lines.) Then my schoolteachers come, all except the history teacher, asking when I'll return to school. I answer, "Tomorrow!"

Lord, what a day, what a celebration! Papa calls around to his friends; all of them are back home. Not all are yet able to move about or even to talk, but all are back home.

Papa went later to the institute. In tears, the director—a remarkable man—Semyon Ivanovich Didenko, embraced him and explained that he had tried as best he could to hold out, but just recently was forced to call a party meeting at which my father was routinely branded an enemy of the people, a murderer, a monster, and thrown out of the party. Didenko was delighted that my father was now free, and Papa told him to forget about the meeting; he understood everything and was amazed at how long the director had managed to hold off the inevitable.

Life gradually returned to normal, and I was back at school. Studying was as natural to me as breathing. Soon my class-mates' burning interest in me cooled, and my life became easier. When Papa returned to work, many of his colleagues could not look him in the eye. And a little later, Lina Stern reentered our life, from prison and labor camp—as the sole survivor of the Jewish Anti-Fascist Committee—this at the age of about eighty. I became very close to her and cherish the memory of meetings and conversations.

April 4th became a traditional holiday in our family. In the first post-Stalin years, twenty-five to thirty survivors of the Doctors' Plot (those who had been imprisoned and others who had waited fearfully) gathered around our table on this day. Their number decreased gradually, as age took its toll; today only my father remains. Yet we continue to celebrate the day— the day of our family's rebirth.

N.R.
Moscow, 1990

– I –

The Conspiracy

ON JANUARY 13, 1953, the world was shocked by the news from Russia. The national newspapers and Radio Moscow disclosed a conspiracy in the Soviet Union (primarily in Moscow), a plot in which prominent physicians were involved. These "murderers in white coats" had caused many deaths by prescribing harmful treatments. Among the victims named were such political figures as Shcherbakov and Zhdanov and some leading generals. The conspiracy, it was alleged, included prominent members of the Soviet medical profession: professors and academicians (subsequently a more humble group of doctors was added to them). Their criminal activities, directed by the intelligence services of various capitalist countries, were not confined to murdering their patients; they were also accused of spying for the same intelligence organizations. The report named several especially active members of the conspiracy—Miron Vovsi, Yakov Etinger, Boris Kogan, Mikhail Kogan, Alexander Grinstein, and others. The list also included Solomon Mikhoels, a famous actor, stage director, and public figure, who had been killed in a hit-and-run accident by a truck several years earlier in Minsk (truck and driver were never found). This criminal plot, it was stated, was based ideologically on Jewish bourgeois nationalism and inspired by an American Jewish organization called Joint. The whole announcement clearly had an anti-Jewish bias.

Even before publication of the report, a number of leading members of the medical profession who were not Jews had been arrested on similar charges—Vladimir Vinogradov, Vladimir Vasilenko, Vladimir Zelenin, Boris Preobrazhensky, Mikhail Yegorov, and a few others. The Jewish group was later complemented by Nikolai Shereshevsky, Mark Sereisky, Yakov Tyomkin, Eliazar Gelstein, Boris Zbarsky, Mikhail Pevzner, Joseph Feugel, Veniamin Nezlin, Naum Wilk, the author of this book, and many more. Some were accused posthumously (Mikhail Kogan and Mikhail Pevzner), while Yakov Etinger had been arrested in 1950 and had died in prison before being included on the new list.

The report published on January 13 was not entirely unexpected. Arrests had begun in November and December of 1952, and, since prominent people were involved, the fact of their arrest could not remain a secret in Moscow and other large cities.

Mass arrests of specialists by profession were nothing new to Soviet citizens. Besides indiscriminate arrests of intellectuals, there had been engineers, civil engineers, career officers, geologists, agronomists, and public figures. In the bowels of the Unified State Political Directorate (OGPU) and its Ministry of State Security (MGB), these individuals were organized into specialized groups of conspirators and subsequently sentenced to death at open or, more often, closed trials. What *was* new about this case were the monstrous charges brought against the medical profession and against physicians of the highest professional standing.

In the history of the Soviet Union, similar accusations had been made against doctors, but these usually concerned only individuals. Chronologically, this list is apparently headed by the surgeon Kholin. He suddenly disappeared in the late 1920s, and no one could imagine what crime could possibly be associated with him. Then rumors leaked out that he had been arrested in connection with the operation for duodenal ulcers which had been performed on Mikhail Frunze, at (it was whispered) Stalin's insistence. On October 31, 1925, after the operation, which was performed by a team of first-class surgeons headed by Ivan Grekov, Frunze died. Rumor had it that Stalin had been instrumental both in subjecting Frunze to the operation and in its fatal outcome. Boris Pilnyak used this plot in his "Tale of the Unquenched Moon," and it was probably this story that cost Pilnyak his life. At the height of the repressions in 1937, he was arrested, charged with spying for Japan (he visited Japan and described his impressions in the book *The Roots of the Japanese Sun*), and shot. Speculation about whether the fatal operation was necessary became rife after Frunze's sudden death and must have reached higher circles, because several days after the funeral, the newspapers published a rather muddled explanation by Chief Surgeon Grekov. Grekov asserted that the operation was necessary and attempted to explain its fatal outcome by insisting that Frunze's health was rather poor in general.

Many of the reports that circulated in Moscow on the cause of Frunze's death (particularly the version of death from an overdose of chloroform anesthesia) were quite plausible medically. But the idea of criminal intent on the part of the surgeons must be rejected categorically, for these were men of impeccable professional integrity. It appears, therefore, that we shall have to be content with the official version of 1925; it is unlikely that further information pertaining to Frunze's death will come to light. (After this book was sent to the printer, however, the editors of the journal *Druzhba narodov* received a letter from Yury Vishnevsky, the son of Konstantin Vishnevsky, a member of the Communist Party since 1919 who was put before a firing squad in September 1941. The letter, prompted by the publication in the journal of excerpts from my book, contains interesting details about Frunze's death which the author learned from his father and which were apparently known to contemporaries close to the tragedy. These details lend additional credence to the suspicions against Stalin.)

We don't know anything about Dr. Kholin's role in Frunze's

operation. If his arrest was in any way connected to it, we may surmise only that OGPU needed him to accuse the surgeons who actually performed the operation, in the event that a case against them might be needed in the future. This was nothing new in the methods of OGPU or the MGB. Very often, minor participants in "crimes" were arrested, and admissions of guilt were forced out of them, while the chief culprits never suspected the danger threatening them. They were not molested but allowed to work and to enjoy a good reputation. The dossiers made up against them often remained unused, since the situation they were prepared for never arose.

Here is one such paradox of Stalin's era that I know about. For many years (from 1926 to 1943) the surgical clinic at the Second Medical Institute in Moscow was headed by Sergei Spasokukotsky. Among his assistants was a certain Dr. Arutyunov, who in 1938 was arrested by the security police and disappeared without a trace. The cause of the arrest was unknown. As an episode all too usual for those times, it was soon forgotten; besides, the man who disappeared was not important enough to pique interest for long. Suddenly, in 1940, the party organization of the institute received a letter from him written on a sheet of ruled paper and obviously posted by somebody who had been discharged from a prison camp. Arutyunov wrote that he had been sentenced to ten years of hard labor for participation in a counterrevolutionary organization allegedly headed by Spasokukotsky. He was sure all those years that Spasokukotsky had been executed, since he, only a rank-and-file member of the "organization" (apparently Arutyunov had been prevailed upon during the investigation to admit to all the charges), had been sentenced to ten years. And then at the camp he had come across a newspaper article with the information that the Presidium of the USSR Supreme Soviet had awarded Spasokukotsky the Order of Lenin. Therefore, not only had the professor not been shot but he was alive and well and looked upon favorably by the government. So Arutyunov was appealing to the party organization of the institute to inter-

26

cede on his behalf as someone who had been wrongly convicted. His plea went unheeded, since nobody at the institute dared question the doings of the MGB: at that time, any doubt as to its infallibility was seen as a crime in itself; if the letter were forwarded to a legal institution, the only result would be fresh reprisals against its author.

A gap of nearly ten years divides the cases of Kholin and Arutyunov, but the similarity of the general pattern makes it clear that the same police methods were still in use. One may be puzzled at the purpose of this concealed discreditation of leading men through minor participants in their fictitious crimes. Apparently, OGPU prepared dossiers against important people "just in case." Informers were not really suitable for the purpose because there had to be some real grounds for gathering and storing information or they would have to be given an assignment to collect such information. The admissions of people at interrogations, no matter how they had been obtained, were regarded as far more convincing. Perhaps, to begin with, Spasokukotsky had not been satisfied with Arutyunov's work and had voiced his displeasure without the slightest ill intent, and some underling took it upon himself to rid a professor, who was highly thought of in upper circles, of an assistant he disliked.

Kholin seemed to be the first test case in the practice of using the medical profession for political purposes. The next case was staggering in its unexpectedness. The victim was Ignaty Kazakov, a doctor with little medical knowledge but much clout. In the 1930s, he proposed "lysatotherapy" as a universal panacea for the innumerable ailments of ageing. It was based on the assumption that all human illnesses are caused by endocrinal malfunctions. It had particular relevance to impotence, a matter of great interest to important political leaders who had entered middle age and whose potency was often undermined by stormy lives and constant stress. To restore the disturbed function of the gland in question, a lysate (a preparation that contained the substance secreted by the gland) was administered to the patient. Only the select few had access to lysatotherapy—major officials, political figures, top military men. A special research institute headed by Kazakov was set up. The institute provided luxurious wards and excellent food for its privileged clientele. Kazakov was immune to normal scientific criticism, having been granted benign indulgence by the nation's leadership.

In her book *The Memory of the Heart* N. A. Rozenel (an actress and the wife of Anatoly Lunacharsky, People's Commissar for Education) recalls how in 1933 her husband, already mortally ill, was visited by his friends, major statesmen, among them Maxim Litvinov, Commissar for Foreign Affairs. They insisted that he should try the method of the miracle-working Kazakov, saying they had themselves been treated by him with amazing results. Kazakov had announced that if Lunacharsky's doctors would allow him to try his method on their patient, he would have Lunacharsky up and about in no time. Persuaded by his friends, Lunacharsky put himself in Kazakov's hands. Before long, however, the healer was caught in an unequivocal sleight-of-hand and refused to continue Lunacharsky's treatment, especially since his cure was clearly having no effect on the dying man.

Knowing about all the favors bestowed on Kazakov, I was greatly surprised by what I was told by Alexei Abrikosov, who in 1934 conducted the autopsy on Vyacheslav Menzhinsky, the head of OGPU. An important OGPU man who was present at the autopsy said to Abrikosov: "See if there are any traces of Kazakov's potion in the body." Abrikosov was amazed not only by the naive suggestion that a pathologist could trace a natural secretion in a corpse but, to an even greater extent, by the implications of the question. At that time, Kazakov was in his heydey. Apparently the sword had already been raised over his head, however, and it would fall four years later.

This means that the charge of malpractice on the part of physicians was already taking shape, to reach full maturity in the trial of 1938, at which physicians were accused of causing the deaths of Maxim Gorky, Gorky's son, Menzhinsky, and others. This trial meted out death sentences to the doctors Lev Levin (employed at the Kremlin Hospital) and Ignaty Kazakov; Professor Dmitry Pletnyov was sentenced to many years' imprisonment and died in a camp. The *Great Soviet Encyclopedia* (1954) has this to say about Menzhinsky's death: "V. R. Menzhinsky died at his post. He was heinously murdered on orders from the ringleaders of the anti-Soviet counterrevolutionary right-wing Trotskyite bloc." (In actual fact, Menzhinsky died of progressive myocardial ischemia, caused by sclerosis of the coronary vessels. Gorky, who suffered from pulmonary disease most of his life, presumably of tubercular origin, died of progressive chronic nonspecific pneumonia with distinct cicatrization of the lungs and a myocardial complication connected with it. No other versions were suggested during the autopsy. It should be noted, too, that all those condemned in the case of the Trotskyites were posthumously rehabilitated in 1988 by special resolution.) The imputation of Gorky's death to his attending doctors, which was put down in the sentence and never openly refuted, was kept alive even after the Doctors' Plot had ended. The scoundrels would not part with their brainchild, as is demonstrated by the following episode.

In 1967 or 1968 (thirty years after the trial in which the story about Gorky's murder by his doctors was concocted), my wife and I were vacationing in the Crimea at the Foros Sanatorium, which belongs to the Central Committee of the Communist Party. There a stupid and conceited young man worked as master of entertainment. Once he took a group of vacationers on an excursion to the neighboring Tesseli Sanatorium, which had been Gorky's summer villa. Trying to impress us with his knowledge, the blockhead showed us a pile of cobblestones and said that the doctors had forced Gorky, under the guise of physical exercise, to carry these stones from one place to another. The strain had supposedly contributed to his demise. The young man was only repeating the myth that was proposed as evidence at the trial of 1938 and was included in the 1954 edition of the *Great Soviet Encyclopedia* (see the entries for Gorky and Menzhinsky); the story had not been publicly repudiated even in the 1967 edition, at least in reference to the doctors' crimes. The sightseers stared with fascinated horror at the pile of stones carried by Gorky's martyred hands.

By the early 1950s, cases of individual "killer doctors" had multiplied, and they were brought together into one mammoth plot involving dozens of the most illustrious names in Soviet medicine. As I have tried to show, the Doctors' Plot was not a bolt from the blue, no meteor from a distant alien world that invaded the atmosphere of our planet. No, it had predecessors and precedents. The phenomenon was the natural fruit of Stalin's regime, and a great deal of conscious effort went into charging the atmosphere until the people's minds were conditioned to accept absurdities. Let us try and work out the principle by which the victims were chosen, at least with respect to two doctors, Levin and Pletnyov.

Lev Levin was a leading doctor in the Kremlin Hospital and an erudite specialist. As a reward for his confession that he had participated in the murder of Gorky and his son, Levin was permitted to write letters to his family from prison. In these notes, using Aesopian language, he managed to give them an idea of conditions in prison, of the charges against him, and the confession wrested from him by threats that his family would be made to pay for his stubbornness. It was to save his loved ones that he had slandered himself.

Levin's eldest son worked at the People's Commissariat for Foreign Affairs. When his father was arrested, he was not in Moscow. Upon his return he wrote a letter to Molotov, asking him to sort out this misunderstanding, since Molotov had been his father's patient and personal friend. He took the letter to the Central Committee personally, and the response to it was immediate: Levin's son was arrested the following night and never heard of again. For many years, Levin's family labored under the misapprehension that the letter had never reached Molotov. But it turned up in the file when Dr. Levin was posthumously rehabilitated. The letter had reached Molotov after all, since it contained a comment written in Molotov's hand: "Why is this 'professor' still at the NKID [People's Commissariat for Foreign Affairs] and not the NKVD (People's Commissariat for Internal Affairs]?" Truly the pun of an executioner! Naturally it had been taken as guidance for further action.

The accusation that Dmitry Pletnyov had killed Gorky and his son appalled the Soviet people, even though after the grim events of 1938 they should have been inured to such hair-raising tales. Pletnyov enjoyed tremendous popularity as a man of science and practicing physician, and he was held in high regard among the Soviet leadership. We still do not know the real reasons behind his arrest and condemnation (he was sentenced to twenty-five years, and much later it became known that he was shot in an Orel prison in September 1941). He probably did not know the reasons himself. There were all sorts of conjectures. Before staging a sensational trial in which the high-ranking Pletnyov was to figure, he was subjected to a vile accusation, aimed at discrediting him as an immoral man. The nature of the slander was characteristic of the crude minds and atavistic imaginations of its authors.

On June 8, 1937, *Pravda* exploded in a denunciation under the hysterical headline, "Professor, Violator and Sadist!" The story told in the article was truly laughable—if one could afford to laugh at absurdities then. It was alleged that a sixty-year-old Professor P. had attacked a female patient B. in a fit of sexual frenzy, bit her several times on the breasts, and thus inflicted a severe physical and moral trauma on her. I knew this woman. She was a reporter for a Moscow newspaper (*Trud*, I believe) and, in my capacity as assistant rector for research and instruction of the Second Medical Institute, I had been obliged to receive her when she sought information for an article. Her appearance was far from glamorous, and it is hard to imagine her arousing any sexual passion. She was about forty, dowdy and unattractive. She always wore a long bedraggled skirt and low-heeled worn-out shoes. She was rather tall, with black, greasy-looking hair and a puffy swarthy face with protruding lips. The only emotion she aroused in me was the desire to be rid of her as soon as possible. And suddenly we were told that she had been the virgin victim of the "lustful" professor, a violator and sadist. I said then that one would only be moved to bite the woman in self-defense, for lack of any other means of protection. Nonetheless, Pletnyov was put on trial for this "barbaric" action and sentenced to two years' imprisonment.

Apparently the whole plot was connected to the suicide of Stalin's wife, Nadezhda Alliluyeva. She shot herself in the temple, though this obvious cause of death was officially suppressed. In the coffin her hair was arranged so as to conceal the gun wound. The official version was death from acute appendicitis, which sounded clumsily improbable even for people not in the know. Those who did know—the head doctor of the Kremlin Hospital Alexandra Kanel, Levin, and Pletnyov—had seen Alliluyeva the day before her death with no signs of appendicitis, and the next morning they saw her in bed, dead, with a gaping wound in her temple and a gun beside the bed. The three of them refused to sign a certificate testifying to death from appendicitis, so it was signed by other doctors. Stalin never forgot or forgave their refusal to comply, and the charge of Gorky's murder was his revenge on Pletnyov and Levin. Kanel died of meningitis in 1936; otherwise she would surely have shared the fate of her two colleagues.

Kazakov's sin against the regime is still a mystery. I have already said that he was received in the top echelons of Stalin's society. Perhaps he knew too many secrets and was not sufficiently discreet. That would have been enough reason for the security men (who had him in their sights, as I have mentioned) to nab him.

— 2 —

Antisemitism

THE ANTISEMITIC overtones of the Doctors' Plot have a long history of preparation and incitement. The campaign against cosmopolitanism launched in 1948 by editorials in *Pravda* and *Kultura i zhizn* prepared the psychological ground. The two editorials accused literary, music, and theater critics, primarily Jewish, of ideological sabotage. These critics, branded as "rootless cosmopolitans," allegedly denigrated works by Russian authors and lauded works alien in spirit to everything Russian and Soviet.

The articles naturally elicited wide response. The critics thus smeared tried to fight back but were crushed by a tidal wave of abuse spouted by numerous sycophants, who readily joined the chase. To characterize the atmosphere, I shall cite from the report on the party meeting held at the Soviet Writers' Union, which was published in *Pravda* on February 11, 1949, under the title "Concerning an Antipatriotic Group of Theater Critics." The speaker was Anatoly Sofronov, secretary of the board of the Writers' Union:

A group of rabid ill-intentioned cosmopolitans, people without kith or kin, mercenary and unscrupulous dealers in drama criticism, have been pilloried in the editorials of *Pravda* and *Kultura i zhizn*. This antipatriotic group has been undermining the foundations of popular culture for a long time. Risen from the rotten yeast of bourgeois cosmopolitanism, decadence, and formalism, the cosmopolitan critics have caused great harm to Soviet literature and art by malevolently smearing and viciously slandering everything that is new and progressive, everything that is best in Soviet literature and theater.

Further on he said: "Yuzovsky, Gurvich, Borshchagovsky, Boyadjiyev, Altman, Varshavsky, Malyugin, Kholodov, and other cosmopolitan antipatriots have taken to their bosoms the ideology of the bourgeois West. They grovel before bourgeois culture, poisoning the wholesome atmosphere of Soviet art with the miasma of bourgeois hurrah-cosmopolitanism, aestheticism, and snobbery." Then Sofronov proceeded to cite examples of their pernicious activities. The malefactors had criticized such patriotic plays as Romashov's *The Great Force* and Surov's *The Green Street*. These plays were produced by the Maly Theater and the Moscow Art Theater and were performed to practically empty auditoriums, although tickets were given out at offices and industrial enterprises free of charge. There were occasions when the theater's manager had to appeal to the audience, on behalf of the actors, to move to the front, since the actors were disheartened by the sight of empty seats. In his report Sofronov virtually annihilated the critic Altman for greeting the production of *Princess Turandot* as a momentous theatrical event (this opinion, by the way, was borne out by the subsequent history of Soviet theater). Subotsky was attacked for "trying to distract the writers' attention from dealing blows to kinless cosmopolitanism." Sofronov also lashed out at the literary critics Ehrlich, Danin, and others. About Danin he said, in particular, that he had inherited the methods of the rabid cosmopolitans who hounded Gorky and Mayakovsky and that he sang accolades to vacuous poets alien to the popular spirit such as Boris Pasternak and Anna Akhmatova (now acknowledged as literary giants). The report was a stream of abuse, which had no regard for even a semblance of truth or for

34

the conventions of criticism or of polite society. Some of Sofronov's vituperations were so elaborate as to defy understanding.

Every social phenomenon must be anchored. So the struggle against the phenomenon of cosmopolitanism had to involve real people, as conveyors of the evil. In the first stage of the campaign, literary critics took the blow. Then signs of cosmopolitanism were sought out in the work of writers and poets. For instance, in Edward Bagritsky's "Ballad of Opanas" the hero is a Jew, Joseph Kogan; and Bagritsky himself was a Jew. In Joseph Utkin's "Story of Red-Headed Motele, the Rabbi Isaiah, and the Commissar Bloch" the title itself is a dead giveaway. These works were proclaimed to be cosmopolitan. In 1965 Ilya Ehrenburg wrote in *Novy mir* about the ordeal to which he was subjected while publishing a five-volume collection of his work. "On almost every page of works that had previously been published many times over, they sought out things which were no longer permissible. Besides various changes in the text, they demanded that I change quite a few names in the stories 'The Second Day' and 'Without Pausing for Breath'." The reproach was that "in these books, written about the Russian people who were, together with other nationalities, building factories and changing the face of the North, there were too many names of persons who did not belong to the basic nationality." There were seventeen such names in "The Second Day" (out of 276) and nine in "Without Pausing for Breath" (out of 174). "I wondered," Ehrenburg writes, "what I was expected to do about the name that stood on the title page." Ehrenburg did not state what "nonbasic" nationality meant (no doubt due to censorship), but it is clear enough from the list of names and the author's own name.

Having no mother country of their own, kinless cosmopolitans, it was averred, were unable to appreciate the work of the Russian people, the nature of things Russian and Soviet, and therefore had no right to pronounce judgments on it. The ideologists of this campaign would have probably forbidden Isaac

Levitan to paint Russian landscapes with his Jewish brush, however brilliant they might have been. In the course of the campaign aspersions were cast on the work of Bagritsky, Svetlov, Vasily Grossman, and many others. The portrait of the composer Felix Mendelssohn was removed from the Grand Hall of the Moscow Conservatory. The portrait of this out-standing nineteenth-century composer, which had been displayed there together with the other composers of world rank, was replaced by one of Dargomyzhsky. Even during Hitler's rule in Germany, it did not occur to anyone to take down the portrait of Richard Wagner at the Moscow Conservatory. That composer was an extreme nationalist who declared that the genius of Beethoven belonged to Germany alone and who was taken by the Nazis to their bosom as the bard of the truly German spirit. Without attempting to compare the standing of Mendelssohn and his substitute, it is worth noting that the public committee which directed the building of the conser-vatory in the nineteenth century decided that only the com-posers of great symphonic music were to be represented in the Grand Hall (Dargomyzhsky did not write a single symphony). Yet Mendelssohn, a German Jew who had survived two auto-cratic emperors of Russia and tsarist antisemitism, was wrested from his place and banished under the auspices of the "struggle against cosmopolitanism."

The ideas behind this struggle are reminiscent of the utter-ings on the nationality question made by Himmler's son-in-law in a dialogue with the Soviet writer Lev Ginsburg (reprinted in *Novy mir*, 1969). This is what the Nazi said: "A nation is a very complicated concept that includes ethnographic, psychological, and biological aspects. And, if you like, racial ones as well. This must be taken into account. I cannot, for instance, accept as a German writer somebody who writes in German but who in origin and biological organization is incapable of expressing the spirit of the nation whose language he uses . . . Of course exceptions are possible, but . . ." At this point Ginsburg asked,

"By an exception you must mean Heine, don't you?" To this the Nazi replied:

> Heine is an extremely contradictory phenomenon. Born on the Rhine and endowed with a very receptive nature, he did assimilate the signs of the German spirit to a considerable degree, which is confirmed by his "Lorelei" . . . Nevertheless Heine never succeeded—and he could not have succeeded—in overcoming his origins, and those of his works where his roots show have remained alien to us . . . Let me cite an example closer to me—the excellent composer Mendelssohn-Bartholdy. Can we regard his splendid music as German? By no account . . . Therefore national culture, like a nation itself, does not tolerate any admixture . . . Only the composition of a person's blood determines to which nation he belongs.

There is no difference between the ideological views held by a fanatical Nazi and the fighters against cosmopolitanism.

Soon, as was to be expected, the struggle against cosmopolitanism and its accompanying "subservience to the west" overflowed the confines of literature and art. The struggle had to be carried on in all spheres of life; cosmopolitans had to be condemned everywhere. The antisemitic slant of this campaign stuck out a mile, and the fig leaf of "Soviet internationalism" did little to conceal it. But the enemies of cosmopolitanism clung to it nevertheless, and the word "Jew" was seldom, if ever, used. But the skimpy fig leaf occasionally proved inadequate, leading to a loss of political virginity. This kind of awkward situation occurred at the Institute of Occupational Diseases. At a sitting of the Academic Council, harsh criticism was leveled at Nikolai Bernstein, a prominent physiologist and author of the excellent monograph *Biomechanism of Movement*, in which patriotically minded orthodox critics had discerned manifestations of subservience to the west. In an attempt to defend her professor, a young graduate student cried out in all innocence: "But it's all a mistake! Nikolai Alexandrovich is not a Jew!" Indeed, Bernstein was a Russian who happened to have a non-Russian name (there are many such people in Russia, who trace their origins to Swedes, Frenchmen, Baltic Germans, and such).

The struggle against cosmopolitanism had nothing to do with the differences in principle between cosmopolitanism and internationalism. At one time, in the works of theoreticians of Marxism, these notions were subjected to analysis and were not found irreconcilably opposed. The struggle against cosmopolitanism organically included condemnation of the west, for its science, culture, literature, and art. Of course the winner in this struggle was proclaimed to be the national Soviet-Russian culture, science, literature, and art. The Soviet people were protected from the pernicious influence of the west not only by propaganda and educational measures but also by a system of restrictions to keep them from western temptations. This system included organized inaccessibility to foreign scientific literature and fiction, the removal of masterpieces of western art from museums and a crusade against its admirers among Soviet artists, and, finally, the propagandizing of Russian classical and Soviet music in opposition to music by western composers. The most fervent fighters against subservience were those unprincipled underlings who ran rife during Stalin's regime and who reviled the west with the same zeal with which they formerly (and afterward as well) bowed to it.

The struggle against cosmopolitanism included fanatical efforts to prove Russia's priority in all discoveries, in the pure and the applied sciences. It is common knowledge that the history of science does not always establish who was the first in a particular field. In any area of science it is possible to trace a spiral of ideas and facts which is crowned by the discovery of a scientific law, the formulation of a scientific theory, or the designing of a completely new type of device. The one who succeeds in synthesizing the information accumulated by predecessors has the legal claim to authorship, not the one who propounded an idea in an abstract or hypothetical form. Scientific foresight, although it sometimes plays an enormous role in scientific progress, must still be developed creatively before it can rank as a discovery. Often, in order to establish priority, it is necessary to conduct a painstaking historical and scientific study if the fact of the discovery has not yet been officially established. The establishment of such priority adds to the treasure trove of national science and deserves to be regarded as a point of national pride.

Unfortunately, in Soviet medicine and biology, the race for priority often assumed the form of an undignified tussle that was an insult to the authentic scientific contributions made by Russians, which were universally acknowledged and never in doubt. Such considerations were beyond the mentality of ignorant claim jumpers. Since there was no need to assert the authorship of such major research as Ivan Pavlov's, the pseudo-patriots concentrated on minor, insignificant achievements, relying on the instructions of Stalin's favorite, the notorious quack Lysenko, to ignore "decaying bourgeois science" as such. The younger generations of physicians and biologists, cut off from the latest achievements in science on an international level, were left to stew in their own juice—the juice of ignorance. Meanwhile, the more enterprising spirits among the pseudo-scientists took advantage of the situation to plagiarize ideas from foreign literature and pass them off as their own original research. In this way, the fighters against "subservience" and for "priority" earned not only patriots' halos but monetary rewards as well.

The hullabaloo about priority in Russian biology and medicine yielded only a few paltry and clumsy claims, which detracted rather than added to the prestige of Russian science. Moreover, many an attempt at restoring "justice" ended in fiasco. The whole medical world, for instance, knows about the microscopic nodes that develop in the tissues of rheumatic patients, especially in the heart. In all international medical literature (including Soviet literature up to then), they were referred to as Aschoff rheumatic nodes, after the German pathologist who discovered and described them in 1904. In 1932 Soviet pathologist V. T. Talalayev described some additional features of these nodes in a monograph in which he himself refers to them as Aschoff nodes. Nevertheless, in the heat of the priorities fight in the late 1940s, somebody had the bright idea of renaming them "Talalayev nodes." Medical researchers who had had no opportunity to study the question, and who were also terrified of any possible accusation of subservience, accepted this change of name without demur, and "Talalayev nodes" inundated Soviet medical literature. Alexei Abrikosov finally had to speak out: he insisted that there were no grounds for the change of name. Still a compromise double name, "Aschoff-Talalayev nodes," came to be used in Soviet medical literature (and nowhere else). Some foreign publications (especially medical studies in East Germany) make a special note that in the USSR Aschoff nodes are referred to as Aschoff-Talalayev nodes. This compromise had at least a semblance of reason, for Talalayev did add to the knowledge of their developmental cycle.

No such justification can be brought forward in two other cases of priority. One concerned the Blumberg symptom of peritonitis known to all surgeons. The zealots of Russian priorities dug up information that this diagnostic symptom was discovered, before Blumberg, by the Russian surgeon Shchetkin; so it was renamed the Shchetkin symptom. The designation was compulsory. It then was established that Blumberg was a Russian professor with a foreign name, so the original name had to be restored. Still, to save face (mainly in the political sense), some occasionally referred to the Blumberg-Shchetkin symptom.

In immunology there exists a phenomenon discovered by the Italian scientist Sanarelli in 1923–24, named after him. Several years later, the prominent Soviet immunologist Pavel Zdrodovsky (a scholar of undoubted integrity) achieved the same effect in a slightly modified form. He made no claim to priority, since the phenomenon he achieved was very close to the original

Sanarelli phenomenon. This did not prevent the priority zealots from ascribing the discovery to Zdrodovsky and renaming it the Zdrodovsky phenomenon (occasionally, as a concession to world scientific opinion, it was called the Sanarelli-Zdrodovsky phenomenon). An article published in the Soviet Journal *Epidemiology, Microbiology, and Infectious Diseases* reported the news in idiotic fashion, according to which Zdrodovsky "had discovered a phenomenon *known as* the Sanarelli phenomenon." The zealots, in their ignorance, could not even cook up a decent-looking sauce for their unsavory dish. This brought to my mind the autobiography of the histologist Khvorostukhin, who was not quite right in his mind. He wrote that in 1916 he discovered formations in the pancreas that some authors refer to as Langerhans islets (they were described by that scientist in 1869).

These examples should suffice to sum up the results of all the hue and cry about Russian priorities in medicine and biology. This did enormous moral damage to the prestige of Soviet science. The campaign ended when the anticosmopolitan movement ended, and today only jokes about priorities have survived. One of them says that, according to reliable data, the law of surplus value was discovered several centuries before Marx by a serf of Saratov province, who failed to publish it because he was illiterate.

Although the priority campaign had petered out by the time the Doctors' Plot was launched, it left a mark on the subsequent history of Soviet medicine. Needless to say, the struggle against cosmopolitanism was not confined to the ideological and political spheres. It also included wholesale expulsions of Jewish professors and lecturers. The list of professors at the Second Medical Institute who were fired included Eliazar Gelstein, Joseph Feugel, Yakov Etinger, Alexander Grinstein, and Anatoly Geselevich, all prominent scientists and highly qualified specialists. With the exception of Geselevich, they were all to be subsequently arrested in connection with the Doctors' Plot. The procedure of expulsion was identical in every case. A commission was appointed to examine the work of the clinic or department headed by the professor in question, and "examiners" also attended his lectures. Predictably, the commission discovered many major defects in his work; the conclusions were discussed at the Academic Council of the institute or only at a party meeting (if the professor was a party member). Then the professor was booted. Not infrequently, the chairman of the investigating commission or some particularly active member of it had a vested interest in the expulsion, because he had been promised the post in question.

The expulsion of Jewish professors from medical schools paved the way for incompetents to obtain responsible posts that they never could have obtained otherwise. Devoid of ability for scientific research, they clutched at the chance to elbow their way up through patriotic baiting of cosmopolitans. Top people in the Ministry of Health could not have been unaware of the detrimental effect the mass dismissal of Jewish specialists was having on the state of medical science, instruction, and health services. But they dismissed these consequences with a shrug—it was a kind of acute disease that had to be outgrown. But then the medical schools of Moscow, Leningrad, and other big cities would be "cleansed" of the Jewish taint. As for successors to the posts that became vacant, they never had a moment's hesitation. The principle formulated by Saltykov-Shchedrin, the great Russian satirist, that brains were conferred together with rank, was obviously accepted by the officials in all seriousness. I shall now describe the hounding of my close friend Eliazar Gelstein.

Gelstein belonged to that generation of physicians who helped put Soviet medical science on its feet in practical and theoretical terms and who trained the army surgeons who acquitted themselves so honorably during World War II. From the very beginning of his medical career, Gelstein demonstrated such brilliant ability as a researcher and organizer that at the age of thirty-four (in 1931) he was offered the department of therapy and the post of director of the Clinic of Internal Diseases at Moscow's Second Medical Institute. He directed the work of this department for twenty-one years (with a break during the war), and his work was highly regarded. By the beginning of World War II Gelstein had earned a reputation as an outstanding clinician. He and I were among the first Soviet medical scientists to volunteer for the Red Army, at the start of the war. He was assigned to the post of chief therapist of the Leningrad Front. There is little need to speak of the immense hardships he had to face during the siege. For this work Gelstein received several government awards and the title of Honored Scientist. Hypertension, a disease that struck many in besieged Leningrad, did not spare him, and he returned from the war suffering from very high arterial blood pressure. After demobilization, he returned to his clinic and his work. He fought his illness bravely and concealed it from the people around him.

Then dark clouds began to gather over his head, the same clouds that were to gather over so many others. An attack in which Gelstein's entire life's work was not merely criticized but demolished was launched by the institute's own newspaper. This was an outrageous lampoon in the usual style of the time. It sneered at his lectures to which, it alleged, students had to be dragged by force; it nullified his administrative record and his research. The proud professor was shattered by this slanderous attack with its brazen distortions of the truth. He took it as a personal insult, failing to discern in it the manifestation of a more general social phenomenon. Events proceeded according to pattern: several of his subordinates (especially an assistant he regarded as his friend) joined in the fray, each casting more or less weighty aspersions on their superior. Gelstein's work was discussed at a party meeting in vociferous and abusive language. At that meeting Gelstein had a severe heart attack. Then followed a discussion of the materials of the investigating commission—which, naturally, confirmed the charges contained in the lampoon and went even further in seeking out more faults. On the morning following that discussion, Gelstein phoned to ask me to come and see him. I never imagined that this proud man could sob so deeply. The wound inflicted upon him could not but tell on his heart, already weakened during the war years. There were more heart problems; a cardiac aneurism developed, and he resigned from his post without waiting for an official dismissal. In 1953 he was arrested in connection with the Doctors' Plot and soon died (in 1955).

I would now like to touch on some events that had a bearing on my inclusion in the group of "murderers in white coats." They are characteristic of the general atmosphere in the medical world on the eve of the Doctors' Plot. There are also a few people I should like to make special mention of.

At Moscow's First Gradskaya Hospital there was a pathologist I shall call Cleopatra G., a young woman of no great intellect and average professional ability, but with considerable drive to make a career for herself. In 1940 she became one of my graduate students, but my supervision of her research was interrupted in the fall of 1941 by the war, and I didn't meet her again until 1945, when I was put in charge of the pathology department at the Gradskaya. Some details of her standing in the department and our relationship need to be clarified, since they have a bearing on the events of 1953.

While I was away at the front (between 1941 and 1945), Cleopatra G. found herself a protector in Boris Mogilnitsky, who undertook to supervise her thesis. He provided a theme that was primitive and scientifically sterile, but it guaranteed an academic degree—according to the demands of the time. Having had a taste of my exactingness, G. wanted to keep Professor Mogilnitsky as her scientific adviser, aware that this promised easier achievement of an advanced degree. This dual relationship created a certain amount of strain in the department.

In the summer of 1951, G. informed me that she had been summoned to the MGB. To this day I don't understand why she saw fit to inform me about the summons—all the more so in that a pledge of secrecy was usually imposed on the person called in. I suppose that she guessed (or knew) why and, guided

44

by her better feelings, wanted to warn me. After her visit to the MGB, when I asked her what it was all about, she said it had been in connection with her mother's obtaining a residence permit in Moscow (she had come from the Ukraine). This could only be an evasion cooked up by the MGB—very probably she had been assigned to watch and report on my activities. For at this point I noticed a change in her behavior. She assumed an independent air and took to disagreeing with me over the findings of autopsies in cases when, in her opinion, death had resulted from malpractice. I spoke about these complications in my relationship with G. to the head doctor of the hospital and my friend, Abram Topchan. Once I even said I would like to get rid of her. To this Topchan, usually a very cool person, whispered in great agitation: "If we so much as lay a finger on her, we won't be working here tomorrow, you understand?" In this way he let me know that, as head of the hospital, he was aware of G.'s role as an MGB informer. Moving ahead of myself, I will say here that all the details of my relationship with Cleopatra G. and the role Professor Mogilnitsky played in them were known at the MGB, which became clear during my interrogations.

I remember one particular conflict with G. that arose during analysis of an autopsy, an incident that was also mentioned during my investigation. The case in question was that of a young woman who had delivered a healthy baby at the obstetrical clinic headed by Joseph Feugel (subsequently one of the accused killer doctors). Several days after her confinement, the young woman developed severe lesions of the brain and died soon after. The post-mortem examination was performed by G., and when I strolled into the autopsy room toward the end of it, I stumbled on the following tableau: on one side of the dissection table, with the corpse of the young woman opened up on it, stood Cleopatra G. in the attitude of an avenging fury and on the other, pale as a sheet, Professor Feugel and several of his assistants in bleak, crushed poses. G. explained the meaning of this dramatic scene to me: she had discovered thrombosis in

45

the veins of the dura mater, which had caused severe disturbances in cerebral blood circulation. She ascribed the thrombosis to sepsis, that is, to puerperal blood poisoning. This conclusion, judging by the reaction of Feugel and his assistants,
was obviously fraught with danger for them all, terrible enough
to reduce them to this abject state.

Puerperal sepsis is an unpleasant occurrence for any maternity ward. Each case will be discussed by a special committee
of obstetricians. The circumstances are minutely examined,
and epidemiological measures are elaborated to prevent the
spread of the infection. Of course this was an emergency, but
not so exceptional as to reduce the doctors involved to such a
state of horror—particularly the head of the clinic, a man of
great experience. As a rule, puerperal sepsis is traceable to some
pathological problem in the body of the woman which existed
before confinement. That infection should be introduced by an
obstetrician through negligence was extremely unlikely. In normal circumstances, an objective and thorough analysis, which
the clinic can only welcome, helps to establish the cause. But in
this case the doctors obviously were not counting on objectivity; the situation was far from normal. Hence the state of
shock, explained by fear of consequences—a fear that was
amply justified by earlier events.

A concerted attack was already being waged against Feugel,
along with many other Jewish professors who headed departments at the Second Medical Institute. The attack was
mounted in the usual way. His accusers endeavored to prove
the professor's incompetence and unfitness for the post, which
he had occupied for twenty years. Besides, he was accused of
conducting unnamed experiments on *Russian* patients which
were detrimental to their health. A certain Professor Z. led the
smear campaign.

It was clear to me that Feugel was in very real danger, so I
was not surprised at his distress. G.'s conclusion concerning
sepsis must have sounded the tocsin for him. To this day I
cannot decide whether her conclusion was the result of igno-

rance alone: no classical signs of sepsis were present either in the clinical picture of the illness or in the autopsy materials. The only discovery at the autopsy was thrombosis in the veins of the dura mater. Lacking the knowledge to explain its development, G. jumped—arbitrarily and groundlessly—to the conclusion that it was caused by sepsis. To make it clear how absurd this conclusion was, I would have to explain the pathology of sepsis and the criteria for diagnosing it on the dissecting table. Since it is very difficult to explain all this in untechnical language, I will simply ask the reader to defer to my half century of experience in pathology and to take it from me on faith: there was no sepsis and never could have been. An analysis of the case history showed that abnormalities in blood composition had been found in this particular patient during pregnancy. These abnormalities caused the development of thrombosis in the puerperal period, which is generally characterized by disturbances in blood coagulation. But Cleopatra G. insisted on her absurd verdict, and this incident was also included in my dossier as evidence of my connivance in the criminal activities of Jewish professors.

As for Joseph Feugel, his fate had already been sealed. His persecutor, Professor Z., received the job as head of the clinic. He saw my defense of Feugel (done with all possible tact, since I knew what I was up against) as a reflection on his own professional ability. At a chance meeting at the Scientists' Club in the autumn of 1952, he expressed his disapproval of my actions—in rather vague and incoherent terms—and in conclusion said: "Just you wait, soon you'll know." He did not say what I would know, but the words were threatening. Indeed I would know, and all too soon. I saw his hand in one of the charges leveled at me after arrest: connivance with the crimes of terrorist doctors and discreditation of honest Soviet scientists.

The incidents I have described were typical for the time. The only possible difference in outcome was whether the professor being baited would have a heart attack or prove to be of stronger mettle. These events naturally created an unhealthy atmosphere in all the medical schools. The Jewish teachers not yet expelled lived in a state of constant fear and daily strain. Many professors, whether Jewish or not, complained that while delivering lectures, they were constantly apprehensive that they might use a phrase that could be misconstrued and give a pretext for accusations of political distortion. There were observers present at lectures whose sole concern was to catch the speaker in some "cosmopolitan perversion." Some secretly brought tape recorders. One especially tragicomical situation arose in this connection.

The dramatis personae in the episode were Abram Charny, head of the department of pathological physiology of the Central Institute of Refresher Courses for Doctors, a very careful man who lived in constant premonition of unpleasantness of some kind or other, and Shabsai Moshkovsky, corresponding member of the Academy of Medical Sciences, head of the department of parasitology at the same institute, and a highly cultured man of impeccable integrity.

One evening in the fall of 1952, the telephone rang in my office and I heard Charny's agitated voice: "Yakov Lvovich, I believe Professor Moshkovsky is a friend of yours?" Moshkovsky had indeed been a family friend for many years. "In such a case," Charny continued, "I must warn you: tread carefully with him—he is a scoundrel and a provocateur." I did not at first believe he was actually speaking of Moshkovsky, so incompatible were his words with what I knew of my friend. So I asked if he really meant the same Moshkovsky, and when he answered in the affirmative, I asked what had happened. Charny said that apparently I had not heard of Moshkovsky's speech at a meeting of the institute's Professorial Council. I had not, but said I couldn't believe that Moshkovsky was capable of any base action. It appeared that Moshkovsky had spoken about the need for tape recorders in lecture halls. I felt easier at heart, for I remembered that Moshkovsky had complained to me that, because there were no tape recorders available, he often forgot interesting ideas that occurred to him in the course of the lecture. I was in complete agreement with him because every lecture, unless it is delivered by rote, is a creative process, which should be recorded. I asked Charny why he classified this request as a provocation, adding that Moshkovsky had often spoken to me about the need for tape recorders, to which Charny retorted: "Why, don't you understand, he wants all lectures to be tape-recorded!" I understood his apprehension then. Pathological physiology is a major theoretical discipline and, with the witch hunting creating havoc in medical theory, almost any statement was suspect and could be declared heretical by self-appointed judges. There were quite a few such inquisitors, even some of professorial rank, who were out to profit from methodological vigilance. The episode appeared amusing to me at the time, although it was indicative of a state of affairs that was not at all funny. Moshkovsky, by the way, was quite disconcerted to learn that his innocent words had received such a sinister interpretation.

I cannot hope to encompass the entire breadth of the political horizon during this period. I have only suggested our awareness of a powerful psychological pressure in the various spheres of public life, which gradually mounted and reached its culmination in the Doctors' Plot. There was the arrest of Academician Lina Stern. There was the routing of the Jewish Anti-Fascist Committee. Their tragic fate—execution on August 12, 1952— became known only in later years. Jewish culture in the Soviet Union was put before the firing squad, its finest representatives physically destroyed. Earlier there had been the tragic death (or rather premeditated and carefully organized murder) of the wonderful actor Solomon Mikhoels. And finally came Slanski's trial in Czechoslovakia, at which anti-Jewish sentiments were openly voiced for the first time: among the allegations was the participation of Zionists in monstrous crimes, their collaboration with the Gestapo, and their role in Julius Fučik's death. There were some physicians in the dock who were accused of prescribing harmful treatments for leading political figures in

49

Czechoslovakia. I remember the impression these accusations made on me. One did not need much foresight to realize that this trial might be a prelude to something along the same lines in our own country. Anyway there could be no doubt that this show had been master-minded outside Czechoslovakia, where antisemitic tendencies had never been strong. The summer and autumn of 1952 were overshadowed by the Slanski trial and the forebodings it aroused.

There were also minor symptoms observable in the world directly around me. As far as I was concerned, the first stark symptom was a telephone call at my flat in Afanasyevsky Lane, in the winter of 1950–51. When I picked up the receiver, a strange husky voice said to me, without a word of greeting and without addressing me by name: "Listen carefully. Don't repeat a word, and say nothing about this to anyone. I am calling from the MGB. Tomorrow at 3 p.m. come to Volkhonka Street, number 3. You will be met." The tone was peremptory, and you can imagine how disturbed I was by this mysterious command. The one thing I knew was that the MGB was not to be trifled with and that I would have to go. I arrived at the house at the appointed hour, and a tall man (I don't remember whether he wore a uniform or a civilian coat) approached and told me to enter a ground-floor apartment, the door to which was right on the street. It looked like an ordinary home and consisted of several rooms.

In one room was a woman who might have been a house-keeper. She was sewing or embroidering and did not give us a glance when we walked past her. I have no idea if this was an ordinary apartment that the MGB rented for business or a special-purpose apartment owned by the MGB. But I was surprised by the homely atmosphere and cosiness. With my companion, who, after he took off his coat, proved to be wearing the MGB uniform with a captain's shoulder straps, I walked to the last room, where our heart-to-heart talk took place. It began with a polite inquiry about my health and some other general questions, to which I gave general answers. I was taut inside, waiting to hear—even with a measure of curiosity—the reason for the invitation. The secret was soon revealed. The captain began to speak about the complicated and alarming political situation of our country, how we were surrounded by enemies on all sides. These enemies, he continued, were also active inside the country, masked and disguised, and, to thwart their treacherous plans, extreme vigilance was called for. It was for this noble purpose that the MGB required my help. In other words, I was being recruited as an MGB informer.

I was at a loss to understand why the choice had fallen on me and what considerations they had been guided by; this I was to understand only at a much later date. From the conversation (carried on, for the most part, unilaterally) I realized that my interlocutor was specially interested in the sentiments of Jews, in conversations between Jews (in what language?), especially those that had a bearing on political problems and attitudes to the United States and Israel.

The position I took in that conversation was not original. It boiled down to this: I was a Soviet person and a party member, and if I ever noticed any suspicious actions I would regard it as my duty to report them to the appropriate bodies without needing to be recruited by their staff. I was not suited for the role he was offering me because I did not have the right character or mentality. Moreover, in my line of duty I had dealings with corpses rather than with living people. I had no access to information that might interest the MGB, and the circle of persons with whom I was in daily contact was limited, mostly consisting of professors of medicine. Even with them I had conversations mainly of a professional nature. Then the captain asked me to name those people. The list contained persons I had direct contact with (Abrikosov, Anichkov, Vinogradov, Lukomsky, Bakulev, Preobrazhensky, Davidovsky) and also my close friends (I could not help mentioning them) Eliazar Gelstein and Alexander Guber. My longstanding friendship with these two was, undoubtedly, well known. The captain wrote the names down. Subsequently, during the investigation of the Doctors'

Plot, this list appeared in my file and I was interrogated about it. The captain also asked me about my status at work and my living conditions, intimating that both could be considerably improved through the help of his organization. To this I gave a point-blank refusal, saying that I was quite satisfied with both. So, as they say in official communiqués, the two sides did not come to any agreement on the matters discussed, and in parting the captain expressed his disappointment and displeasure.

I supposed that the matter was closed and I would not be bothered again. But I underestimated the persistence of the MGB. Nor did it occur to me that they would not only resort to tempting offers but would also try intimidation—which they did soon enough.

Some time after this meeting, there was another telephone call, and the familiar husky voice invited me to come to the vestibule of the Moscow Hotel at 4 p.m. the next day, where he would be waiting for me at the newsstand. I tried to decline the invitation, saying tomorrow was a busy day at the institute, but the captain said he would arrange with the director that I should be let off. He understood only too well that I would much prefer to make my own arrangements, without intercession from the MGB. I went to this second meeting armed with the experience of the first and fully determined to refuse all offers, even if threatened with arrest. I decided that I must impress on them—beyond a shadow of a doubt—my refusal to inform. So I would be outspoken and would not resort to dodges and evasions, such as a promise to think it over and the like. I realized that if I left them so much as a chink, they would squeeze their way through. I was quite prepared to be arrested then and there, never to come home from the rendezvous.

At the newsstand, the same captain met me and told me to follow him. We entered an elevator, got out at some floor or other, and I was led into a room where a man wearing the uniform of an MGB colonel was waiting for me. The conversation ran along the same lines, but there was less double-talk. The colonel made no bones about needing information about

Jews, specifically about their anti-Soviet moods and intentions, and made it clear that what they wanted from me was not patriotic amateur efforts but a properly regulated activity. The colonel spoke in a harsh tone. He said that they wanted to know, for instance, what was discussed at supper in the intimate circle of one director of a coal trust. He mentioned the name of the director, a Jewish name I had never heard and forgot at once. Perhaps his post was different, but I remember distinctly that it had to do with coal. I refrained from asking how they expected me to get an invitation to supper from a person I didn't know (and who didn't know me). Such a question, I realized, would provide them with that very chink I was so wary of. They would simply promise to arrange an invitation from the "coal man" for me. The colonel had before him the list of people I had steady contact with—the one the captain had taken down at our first meeting—and coming upon the name of Guber, he said they wanted me to sound him out. I told them Guber was not a doctor but an art critic, to which the colonel replied that he was interested in art critics too. I then added that Guber was not a Jew but a Russian, after which the colonel's interest waned.

The conversation turned to Israel and the Jews' dreams of going there to live. I said I knew nothing about any such dreams, at least I had never heard those sentiments from the Jews I knew, but if there were those who wanted to go, in my opinion, they should be allowed to, for the Soviet Union did not need them. To this the colonel replied, "No, we cannot permit it." Gradually the colonel's tone, initially calm though hostile, became excited, almost violent. After I said that I was not made for the role of an informer and had never heard any incriminating utterances from the Jewish scientists in my circle, the colonel asked me point-blank: "You mean you never heard it said by Jewish scientists that their heads are no worse than those of American scientists, but that their work is inferior to the Americans'?" I felt a chill creep down my spine. These were my own words, and I had said them to my roommate in the

Istra Sanatorium in the previous winter of 1949–50. I had been talking about research in the USSR, its poor organization and the consequent low efficiency, despite considerable outlays, and I did say that our heads were no worse than those of American scientists. Hearing this sentence from the colonel, taken out of context by the informer (clearly my roommate at the sanatorium), I realized that this was the ax they would hold over my head to force me to agree to their proposal. I pretended to be unaware of the anti-Soviet interpretation that could be applied to these words and said they testified only to the speaker's patriotism and concern for Soviet science. The colonel responded with an obscenity and the order, "Get the hell out!" to which I readily complied, taking with me dire presentiments about the prospects for Jews—such interest in them, or in nationality in general, in the year 1950 boded no good.

The episode of my recruitment did not stop there. It ended only in the spring of 1951, when I was summoned to a military registration office somewhere in Sretenka Street, which is in close proximity to the dread Lubyanka Prison, the MGB head office, and not in the district where I was actually registered. I said nothing to my wife but decided that, if I suddenly disappeared, she must be told what had happened to me. I took my modest savings to a family of close friends, warning them that I might not return from my visit to the military registration office and asking them to help my wife should this happen. In a big empty room at the so-called registration office, I found a young man who read me a statement of my refusal to cooperate with the MGB and a pledge of secrecy about the conversations I had had with its representatives. I signed the paper without hesitation. The recruitment episode cropped up again during the investigation of the Doctors' Plot.

By quoting my own words, the MGB colonel had given me to understand that they had an eye on me not only as a potential informer but also as a potential suspect. Many Soviet people had to live with this threat hanging over them. It was pushed into our subconscious, but alarm signals were sounded every

54

time we learned of yet another victim. The great adaptability of the human psyche, however, made possible peaceful coexistence with this fearsome menace. Everyday work, professional, creative, and family concerns, all helped us to forget. To myself, and occasionally in the company of trusted friends, I cited an ironic line from Pushkin's *Boris Godunov:* "The life of Boris' men is to be envied." The certainty of a final end to one's existence does not prevent one from enjoying life, from savoring a taste for it. If anything, this is even accentuated by the premonition of danger. I gradually relegated the chill breath of the Lubyanka to some backyard of memory, and it only surfaced occasionally as a kind of memento mori—a reminder about the inevitability of death, a Latin phrase some lugubrious wit translated as "don't forget to die."

− 3 −

Pathology

IN THE SUMMER of 1951, the Institute of Morphology, which had been under the auspices of the Academy of Medical Sciences, was closed down as a "nest of Virchowianism." Many of its employees, particularly Jews, found themselves unemployed. As for me personally, the laboratory I headed at the Institute of Morphology was located on the premises of the First Gradskaya Hospital's pathology department, which was also in my charge. So after the institute closed, I was left with the hospital job. Soon I took a second post at the Tarasevich Institute as head of the laboratory of pathomorphology, in keeping with my professorial rank. In these two capacities I worked until my arrest on April 3, 1953. I would like to describe the atmosphere at both establishments, since they were directly connected with the events leading up to my arrest.

I shall begin with the First Gradskaya Hospital, one of the oldest and largest hospitals in Moscow. For many decades, since the beginning of the century, this hospital served as the proving grounds for the clinics of the Second Medical Institute (originally the Higher Medical Courses for Women; later the medical department of the Second Moscow University). These clinics were always headed by noted medical scientists, who set the standards for medical treatment, research, and education. Thousands upon thousands of doctors were trained in these clinics and later cherished the memory of their instructors.

During my time, prominent among the professors were the therapeutists Vladimir Vinogradov (replaced at the end of the 1940s by Pavel Lukomsky), Eliazar Gelstein, and Yakov Etinger; the surgeons Sergei Spasokukotsky and Alexander Bakulev (who replaced him in 1943); the eye specialist Mikhail Averbakh; the neuropathologists Lazar Minor and Alexander Grinstein; the otolaryngologists Sverzhevsky and Boris Preobrazhensky; the gynecologists Isaac Graude and Joseph Feugel. All these doctors were outstanding clinicians and teachers, and when most of them became victims of the Doctors' Plot, the hospital was deprived of its finest talent. An irreparable loss was sustained by Soviet medicine.

The head doctor of the Gradskaya Hospital was Abram Topchan, who simultaneously directed the Clinic of Urology and, starting in 1937, was also rector of the Second Medical Institute. Topchan was a veteran party member and a kindly, good-natured person, remarkable for his tact. He enjoyed great popularity among his students and deep respect among his peers. He was dismissed from all his posts, one by one. In 1951, when the dismissal from the last post (rector of the Second Medical Institute) was prepared, they could not find a suitable pretext. He was no longer working, and his job was already occupied by former Deputy Minister of Health for Personnel Milovidov. So a brief announcement appeared in the newspaper *Meditsinsky rabotnik* (Medical Worker), which carried no explanation for the dismissal: "Director of Moscow's Second Medical Institute, Professor Abram Borisovich Topchan, has been dismissed from his post."

Working among these killer doctors, the MGB reasoned, I certainly could not resist the temptation to get involved with them and contribute my fair share. Here I would like to explain the functions of pathologist in a hospital and his relationship with clinicians, the main "culprits in the crime," so that the reader can trace the logic behind the Doctors' Plot. Otherwise it will not be clear how a post-mortem pathologist could be accused of murder.

The pathology department is to a large extent the center of

the entire hospital and is directly connected with all its clinical departments. These are very sad connections because they all come together at the deathbed, something that anyone dealing with diseases has to face. Autopsy is the final stage in establishing the diagnosis. Any death, unless it is a natural death of old age, is in some sense a defeat for the medical profession. So one of the tasks of the pathologist is to establish whether everything possible had been done for the patient. This is a difficult task in every case, requiring a high degree of professionalism and total objectivity on the part of the pathologist.

The aim of an autopsy is to establish whether the diagnosis was correct. The pathologist examines whatever changes he finds in the organs and compares them with the patient's case history, thereby determining to what extent the post-mortem diagnosis differs from or coincides with the clinical diagnosis. If the difference is great, it means there was an error in diagnosis. Not infrequently, lengthy microscopic tests of organs and tissue specimens are required. These also help to establish whether the treatment was suitable, appropriate to the disease, as established by the autopsy. This is particularly important whenever surgery has been involved, and the pathologist may find himself in a very delicate situation. Only in cases of very serious errors in the initial clinical diagnosis can the pathologist draw any conclusions about how much the error affected the treatment and whether proper treatment was not given as a result. However, even then, such a conclusion cannot be made unilaterally. The traditional procedure for pronouncing such judgments is for the pathologists and clinicians to get together and discuss all the information contained in the case history and all the data obtained during the autopsy. Medical control commissions are set up to study all the material pertaining to the patient, including the autopsy data concerning the nature and essence of the error in the diagnosis or treatment, if any has been found.

A "medical error" has been defined as "conscientious delusion on the part of a physician." The word "conscientious" is very important here. It is assumed that the doctor has done everything possible in the line of duty; he has applied all his knowledge to make the diagnosis and prescribe treatment, but nevertheless committed an error that is later discovered during the post-mortem. Carelessness resulting in a medical error is qualified in different terms: as a criminal error or as clinical negligence. My experience shows that even the greatest competence and professionalism do not guarantee perfect diagnoses—they only increase the possibility of such a guarantee. The short duration of the patient's stay in the hospital (owing to belated hospitalization) and the gravity of the condition may prove to be beyond modern diagnostic capabilities, especially in the absence of up-to-date medical technology based on the latest achievements in electronics, automation, radio isotopes, and so on. But even when this powerful technical arsenal is available, the doctor's mind still remains the major factor. The doctor should be able to analyze the symptoms and information obtained in medical examination and to arrive at the diagnosis by synthesizing this information. Even the most sophisticated computer cannot replace the doctor's mind. As methods of diagnosis improve, greater accuracy is expected in diagnosing illness. During the last decade, highly sophisticated test methods have been made available to medicine. The development of cardiac, vascular, and brain surgery has created a demand for greater accuracy in testing. This applies primarily to medical establishments specializing in the treatment of particular diseases or diseases of particular organs.

To be able to conclude that a medical error has been made with any degree of accuracy, the pathologist must, apart from possessing specialized knowledge, take into account the clinical picture and all the details pertaining to the patient's care and diagnostic tests. The pathologist is not usually expected to make a final judgment as to the correctness of the treatment given, except in cases of obvious and impermissible errors, such as surgical errors. His task is to ascertain the absence of the treatment indicated or the presence of a contraindicated treatment for a particular disease. But even this requires considerable acumen and careful formulation of criticism, unless it is to resemble that amusing vignette from Chekhov's notebook: "The patient died because he was given sixteen drops of Valerian instead of fifteen." Medication varies for one and the same disease depending on the form it takes, the stage, and the doctor's experience in treating the disease and using one medicine or another. The assortment of medicines available changes constantly because the effectiveness of various drugs is reevaluated from time to time. At doctors' conferences, heated arguments often flare up among specialists, all of whom are authorities in their fields, regarding the use of a certain drug and the treatment of a particular patient. Opposing views on one and the same method of treatment are often voiced.

And yet it was precisely the accusation of "premeditated incorrect treatment" that figured in the Doctors' Plot, while the obliging experts from the MGB readily supported versions of incorrect treatment in much the same terms as Chekhov's satirical line quoted above. There is a humorous story, well known in medical circles, about a famous clinician from Vienna, Professor Eppinger, who once examined a private patient and discovered an incurable disease. As an honest doctor, he predicted a fatal outcome within a year. Several years later, quite by chance Eppinger met that same patient in good health and was genuinely surprised that his prediction had not come true. He asked about what had been done for him and then commented: "You were given the wrong treatment." Perhaps this is only a joke, although some say it did actually take place. In the period I am talking about, any anecdote, however ludicrous, could easily be turned into horrible reality, a criminal version of intentionally incorrect treatment.

Since ancient times, pathologists have been dissecting corpses to perform post-mortem examinations. For many centuries, the pathologist had to rely on his own power of observation and keen vision to establish the nature of the disease, but always in accordance with current notions. These notions were constantly changing and continue to change today as methods of testing develop and become enriched by achievements in related sciences, particularly microbiology, virology, biology, genetics, and technological progress in general. The electron microscope has become a powerful weapon in the hands of the pathologist. It allows him to study the elements of a cell only several Angströms in size (one Angström is equal to a hundred-millionth of a centimeter), that is, to distinguish the molecules that compose a cell.

Thanks to the introduction of the electron microscope, biopsies of living tissues have become widespread. This has improved the work of physicians, surgeons, and pathologists considerably, making possible early and more accurate diagnosis. Performance of diagnostic biopsies (examination of specimens specially extracted for diagnostic purposes) is the heavy responsibility of the pathologist. His conclusion will determine the general diagnosis and the corresponding treatment. For example, if a woman has a tumor in the mammary glands, it is necessary to determine if it is benign or malignant. In the first case it is enough to remove the tumor while, in the second, radical surgery is required (resection of the whole gland with the adjacent soft tissue of the breast, the nearby lymph nodes, and sometimes even the removal of the ovaries), as well as subsequent chemotherapy and radiation therapy. Thus the pathologist's conclusion is decisive in a vitally important question: the need for a relatively harmless, mild operation or an extensive resection.

Performing diagnostic biopsies and examining surgically removed organs is as much part of the pathologist's work as is dissecting corpses. The pathologist often endures great mental anguish because of his responsibility for human life, particularly when the microscopic picture of a biopsy is not clear and it is difficult to make a definite diagnosis. Additional consultations with colleagues are invariably sought so that the most accurate judgment can be reached.

This brief description of the role of the pathologist by no means exhausts the subject. I made no mention of the extensive research work carried out. But even this short account gives some idea of the pathologist's complex, varied, and highly responsible duties, requiring extensive knowledge of clinical pathology in all fields, constant study, and accumulation of experience. In no other medical branch is there such wide use of group consultation.

I consider this introduction necessary because the Doctors' Plot did involve medicine, and it was put into the hands of evil-minded scoundrels who were completely incompetent to appraise a doctor's actions. Moreover, they did not even attempt to be objective, since that would have prevented them from carrying out the political liquidation that was their real purpose.

- 4 -
Drug Control

THE SITUATION described above refers mainly to my work as a clinical pathologist at the First Gradskaya Hospital. The atmosphere at the Tarasevich Institute of Control of Medicinal Preparations was quite different. I had been connected with the Tarasevich Institute since 1947, first as a consultant on pathological morphology. In 1951 I took a permanent position there. It was one of the first institutes to be set up in the Soviet Union. It specialized in purely microbiological problems, and its task was to test various drugs and antibacterial serums and vaccines before they were introduced on a wide scale. Every year many new drugs are made available to medicine, and the Tarasevich Institute was responsible for checking the quality of all the medicinal preparations made in the nation. The institute checked not only the newly invented drugs but also each series of a new drug already being mass-produced. (Today the organization is known as the Scientific Research Institute for Standards and Control of Medicinal Preparations.)

Soviet scientists have made a sizable contribution to the preparation of new vaccines and serums. Many of them had to pay with their lives for the privilege. I do not mean to say that they became infected while working with actively virulent organisms in their laboratories, although such cases have been known. Those scientists never used themselves as guinea pigs

63

to check their most daring hypotheses or to stage their most dangerous experiments, though the history of science knows such heroes too. No, Soviet scientists fell victim to the virulent activities of the OGPU-MGB, which mowed them down much more effectively than the deadliest of epidemics. At one time microbiology was the focus of their attention, and the first victim, chronologically, was the Mechnikov Institute headed by a major microbiologist, Stepan Korshun.

In 1930, Korshun and a number of his colleagues were arrested. Some of them were later released, but Korshun died in a prison camp. The next large group of major microbiologists was arrested in the years of mass repression (1937–1939). This included Barykin, Krichevsky, Gartokh, Velikanov, and other fine scientists responsible for major contributions to microbiology. They were all accused of anti-Soviet activity and sabotage in their specific fields. Naturally they confessed to their crimes and were duly punished—death by firing squad. Barykin developed a vaccine that is still produced and still bears his name. Krichevsky was the founder and first director of a major research institute of microbiology that covered a wide range of problems and trained an important school of highly qualified microbiologists. He confessed that he organized the institute for the purpose of carrying out acts of microbiological sabotage. Lyubarsky, an authority on the microbiology of tuberculosis, must have decided that the more absurd his evidence was, and the wider the circle of microbiologists allegedly involved in criminal activities, the more obvious the sheer idiocy of the accusations against him would be. But he reckoned without the host. OGPU officials welcomed any absurdity as long as it provided a pretext for capital punishment. Accusations against other microbiologists were of much the same nature, and all sentences were passed without consulting expert opinion. Instead, the dossiers of the accused microbiologists contained slanderous denunciations by incompetents out to further their own careers. (When these microbiologists were rehabilitated posthumously, the procurator's office sent their dossiers to the

Tarasevich Institute for expert opinion on the materials of the case. As an employee of the institute, I had access to these materials.)

Among those arrested were such major scientists as Lev Zilber and Pavel Zdrodovsky, but they were forced to work in their fields while in prison, under the supervision of OGPU people; they were later released and reinstated. Arrests among bacteriologists which swept the country constituted, in actual fact, the routing of Soviet microbiology as a science on the eve of an already imminent war, with the threat that the bacteriological weapons being developed in many countries along with defenses against them might actually be used. In whose interest was the elite of Soviet microbiology destroyed at that particular time? In whose interest were the generals and scientists liquidated? These questions still remain a mystery of the Stalin era.

Here is one episode connected with the arrests of microbiologists in 1937. At the time I had contacts with Medgiz Publishers, both as author and editor. The head of Medgiz was David Weiss, a firm and experienced manager. His editor-in-chief, Severin Weinberg, an astute and enthusiastic man, was in love with the publishing business and science. Both of them fell victim to Stalinist repressions and disappeared without a trace. They were probably arrested on individual charges not connected with their publishing activities. The new Medgiz director, a middle-aged woman whose name I can't recall, was quite ignorant of medicine and in general an uncultured person, a typical product of those times.

Soon after the change in management, Medgiz sent the proofs of a manual on microbiology to the author, Professor Yeliseev of the Ivanovo Medical Institute. The proofs were sent with the usual request that they be reviewed and promptly returned with the author's signature. When no proofs arrived by the appointed deadline, the editors sent two telegrams to Yeliseev—again no answer. The third telegram brought the proofs back, without the author's corrections, accompanied by a short letter from his wife saying that Yeliseev was ill. Illness seemed to be spreading among microbiologists everywhere. Should suspicions be confirmed, the publication of the book had to be stopped and the name of its author consigned to oblivion. But how was one to get this confirmation? If the suspected arrest turned out to be hearsay, one could get into trouble for spreading false rumors. Even if it were true, one dared discuss it only in whispers in order not to mar the general cheerful atmosphere. The new Medgiz director found a happy way out, she thought, by sending a telegram with what appeared to be a sufficiently cryptic message: "Cable if Yeliseev is ill or something else." There was no answer, but later we learned that it was the fateful "something else." Yeliseev disappeared into the dungeons of the OGPU-MGB, and not a word has been heard of him since. Among those associated with Medgiz, the phrase "something else" came to be used symbolically.

At the Tarasevich Institute, my job was to test the quality of vaccines and serums. Animals, such as guinea pigs, rabbits, white mice, and rats (and in certain cases monkeys, for testing polio vaccine), were inoculated with the preparation being tested, and then a morphological examination of the animal's organs was done to reveal the presence or absence of pathological changes. No changes were considered proof of its harmlessness. The morphological test also enabled us to establish the vaccine's capacity for creating immunity.

Head of the Tarasevich Institute then was S. I. Didenko, a man of peasant origin who had been through the mill. He spent World War I in the Black Sea navy. Upon graduation from a military medical school, he served as a doctor's assistant on the cruiser *Prut*. After the civil war in Russia was over, he was able to complete his education and get a medical degree. Later he specialized in microbiology and defended his graduate thesis after I was already working at the institute. The institute's party organization was relatively numerous: some twenty persons, mainly women (the staff was also predominantly female). Most of them were intellectuals of the Stalinist brand, narrow specialists (some of them with high academic degrees), individuals of little culture, robots who unquestioningly accepted the fanatical cruelty of Stalin's regime. They would just as readily have hailed fascism had it been presented to them as communism. In all fairness, it must be mentioned that later, after the revelations at the Twentieth Party Congress, many of them revised their views and publicly admitted that they had been wrong.

My research at the Tarasevich Institute was crowned by the development of a general theory of morphological processes in animals inoculated with various vaccines. By connecting all the complex cellular processes, I formulated the theory of immunomorphology as a new branch of immunology. The theory of immunomorphology in general and special pathologics of infectious and certain other diseases were later developed by my followers, and I was recognized as the founder of the theory not only in the Soviet Union but in other countries as well.

When I took the job at the Tarasevich Institute, in the fall of 1951, I joined its party organization and soon became aware of a split in its ranks. There was also a small vacillating group of centrists. The tense atmosphere in the outside world naturally affected our microworld. In the fall of 1952, a sinister rumor was circulated among the institute's staff to the effect that Rapoport had signed up for a season ticket to the Jewish Theater. This rumor, invented by the local party leadership, was repeated in whispers, and the reaction was one of horror, as if I had murdered a child or worse. Actually, the sale of such season tickets had been announced quite openly in the press, so there was nothing criminal or illicit about buying one. The purpose of issuing the tickets was to attract wider audiences, since attendance had fallen off sharply. Jews themselves were afraid to be associated with this center of Jewish culture, which was already marked by terror—the arrest of the theater's leading actor, Zuskin (he was executed in August 1952), and the hit-and-run murder of Mikhoels, the theater's life and spirit. Neither the

murderers nor the reasons for Mikhoels' death have been uncovered. But no one had any doubts that the murder was somehow connected with the terror emanating from the MGB
building in Dzerzhinsky Square (formerly Lubyanka). Any
contact with Jewish culture through this theater became if not a
sign of Jewish bourgeois nationalism, at least a pretext to suspect a person of such sentiments, which was the equivalent of
being suspected of anti-Soviet activities and counterrevolutionary intentions; that in turn was but one step from treason and
espionage. No wonder the Jewish population of Moscow came
to fear its own theater, which was then playing to a practically
empty house. To all appearances, the theater still existed and
was supported by the state, but in actual fact it turned into a
"thing in and of itself," avoided by the very people it existed
for. It was rumored, probably without grounds, that anyone
who went there was shadowed from then on and was registered
at the MGB as a potential enemy of the Soviet Union. The
rumor, for whatever its worth, was typical of the atmosphere of
those days.

When the rumors of my buying a season ticket for that offen-
sive, albeit quite legitimate, theater reached the vigilant party
cell to which I belonged, I became automatically suspect. Our
local party leaders had enough prudence not to discuss this
piece of gossip with me (though I learned about the whole thing
from our party secretary), for that would have been too obviously antisemitic. So their reaction was limited to malicious
gossip. In reality, I never bought a season ticket. Since I knew
very little Yiddish, I seldom went to the Jewish Theater. I only
went to see the plays I knew (such as *Travels of King Benjamen III*
or *King Lear*, to name just two) to admire the remarkable acting
of Mikhoels, Zuskin, and others. I did not really follow the
activities of the theater and did not even know about the season
tickets being issued to save it—otherwise I would have bought
one.

In the fall of 1952, I became aware of an outside interest in my person. A special commission was appointed (as far as I remember it represented, officially, the Moscow Party Committee) to inspect the quality of the institute's scientific personnel. Soon it became obvious that they were only interested in one member of the staff—me. Their talks with the others were only a cover. From my first conversation with the chairman of the commission (the other members never showed up), I understood what they wanted of me. My inspector was a man of about forty-five or fifty, well-educated, and quite presentable. At least his speech was reasonably literate. He was dressed in a military tunic without shoulder straps and could have been taken for a recently retired officer.

The inspector inquired about members of my laboratory and was apparently satisfied to find them Russian. At that time I had only two people working under me: Tatyana Migulina and a rather listless graduate student who shall remain nameless (more about her later). Migulina had been a student in my class at Moscow University. She had no special talent for research, which later became evident from her career. Her abilities were only sufficient to make a competent laboratory assistant, and at this level she remained all her life.

The inspector was interested in the substance of our research. He could not understand what morphological analysis had to do with vaccine and serum quality control, so I had to go into lengthy explanations. He was particularly concerned about the training of the people in my laboratory, despite the paucity of their number. What were my plans for Migulina, he demanded to know. I thought I should display the proper spirit in light of the general tendencies of the times and said that I was planning during the next six months to prepare the young woman to take charge of the laboratory (though she had none of the essentials for such a position), so that it wouldn't remain without a head when I was dismissed. This plan met with his enthusiastic support, and he couldn't help exclaiming "That's right!" forgetting that the author of the plan was also its victim.

Perhaps he had not forgotten anything but thought it quite natural for a Jew to show some spirit of self-sacrifice for the common good. At any rate, he took my bait and revealed the aim of his inspection. I later recounted this story in a bitter and ironic vein to our director: Didenko shared my bitterness but not my irony.

– 5 –

Gathering Clouds

THE YEAR 1952 was about to start. We were aware of a marked thickening of the political and social atmosphere, a thickening oppression that was nearing the point of suffocation. The feeling of alarm, the premonition of dire and inevitable disaster, achieved a nightmare intensity at times, supported, moreover, by actual facts. In December 1950, Yakov Etinger and his wife were arrested. Their arrest was preceded by the mysterious disappearance of their adopted son Yakov, a student at Moscow University. One day he left for the university and never returned. Etinger was at his wit's end. He appealed to prominent workers of the MGB who were his patients to help him search for the young man, who, he feared, might have been lured out of the city and murdered. His powerful patients assured him that everything possible was being done, but so far they had failed to trace his son. As was to be expected, Yakov was then being held in prison, arrested by MGB men on his way to the university. In the vernacular of the MGB, such an action was termed "secret lifting," and its purpose in that particular case was quite unfathomable, unless it was motivated by the sadistic desire to cause additional mental suffering to the family. On the very eve of Etinger's arrest, I visited him and found him extremely depressed. Over the next few days, I phoned him several times to find out if he had learned anything about Yakov's whereabouts, but there was no answer. This was sinister, and very soon my fears were confirmed. More disappearances followed. All the members of the Jewish Anti-Fascist Committee—writers, actors, and scientists—were arrested, never to be seen again. Then the scientist Lina Stern disappeared. In the summer of 1952 many outstanding doctors who had worked in the Kremlin Hospital for many years and treated many statesmen were summarily fired. Among them were Miron Vovsi and Vladimir Vinogradov. The former head of the Kremlin Hospital, Alexei Busalov, Mikhail Yegorov, Yakov Etinger, and Sophia Karpai were arrested. The work of Academician Alexei Abrikosov and his wife Fanny Abrikosova-Wulf (a pathologist), and many others, was cut off.

I make no claim to the role of historian of the Doctors' Plot. I have had no access to relevant documents. Also I was not directly connected with the center of the activities of the killer doctors—the Kremlin Hospital. Information about alarming events there reached me from time to time, but then (and later too) to show any interest in such events was decidedly unhealthy. However, even those who worked in that hospital, if they dared at all to talk to me about the sinister goings-on, confessed to utter perplexity.

Later I learned that the first pathologist to be arrested at the Kremlin Hospital was Anatoly Fyodorov. He was subsequently released, but I soon lost track of him and therefore know nothing about what charges were brought against him (I suppose they were the standard ones) or how his life continued in later years.

A minor but characteristic detail of the period: my elder daughter Naomi, who graduated from the Second Medical Institute in 1952, was assigned to work in the MGB system on Sakhalin Island—that is, to be a doctor in a concentration camp. She dared not demur. I realized that this was the kind of job that could perhaps be handled by a hefty man but not by a young woman and, believing that the appointment had to do with the person of her father, tried to intercede with Deputy

Minister of Health Alexander Shabanov. After hearing my story, Shabanov blurted out: "Really, that's too much!" Naomi was reassigned to Velikiye Luki, a town in Central Russia, but the personnel director of the Ministry of Health changed the assignment to Toropets, a smaller town in the same region. That was where my daughter went to work after her graduation.

Autumn had come—the last autumn of Stalin's regime. Events were mounting to a climax. Horrible news was passed by word of mouth. The MGB had disclosed a Jewish conspiracy at the Moscow automobile plant. Mass arrests had been made, wreaking havoc on the leading engineering and technical personnel. Attempts of the plant's director, Likhachev, whose name the plant now bears, to intercede for his engineers were fruitless. More Jewish plots were uncarthed—in the Moscow Metro and elsewhere. Sinister rumors crept about Moscow, which it was difficult (and dangerous) to try and check. It was said that Vovsi, Kogan, Vinogradov, and Feldman had been arrested. One dared not try and check—even uttering their names aloud was dangerous. We had to pretend that nothing untoward was happening. But gradually confirmation of the rumors did arrive. Vinogradov's son Vladimir (subsequently a professor of surgery) was an assistant of Alexander Bakulev, head of a clinic in the First Gradskaya Hospital. Once Vladimir came to my pathology department on business. He looked dejected, and I ventured to ask him, "How are things with your father?" He curtly replied, "Bad." So it *was* true. One professor of medicine after another was arrested (Vasilenko, Grinstein, his wife Popova, Preobrazhensky, Yegorov, and many others). The medical world was not simply deflated, it was crushed. Nobody knew anything for certain, but it was clear that yet another exposure of a conspiracy was in the offing—this time among the top men in the medical profession—and everyone in that group who was still at large expected arrest each night. I remember our New Year's celebration of 1953 among close friends. The mood was far from festive. Everyone was apprehensive of what the new year would bring, and of course no one had an inkling of the ultimate liberation that was in store for us all. I made a toast to freedom—in its concrete, not its philosophical, meaning.

Then came the memorable day of January 13, 1953. The storm finally broke. The Tass news agency published a government statement, which I shall quote verbatim:

> January 13, 1953. From the latest news.
> Arrest of a group of subversive doctors.
> Some time ago, the bodies of State Security uncovered a group of terrorist doctors who set themselves the task of cutting short the lives of prominent public figures in the Soviet Union by administering harmful treatments.
> This terrorist group includes: Professor M. S. Vovsi, a therapeutist; Professor V. N. Vinogradov, a therapeutist; Professor M. B. Kogan, a therapeutist; Professor B. B. Kogan, a therapeutist; Professor P. I. Yegorov, a therapeutist; Professor A. I. Feldman, an otolaryngologist; Professor Y. G. Etinger, a therapeutist; Professor A. M. Grinstein, a neuropathologist; G. I. Maiorov, a therapeutist.
> Documentary data, pathological investigations, conclusions of medical experts, and admissions of the culprits have established that the criminals, who were covert enemies of the people, prescribed incorrect treatments and so undermined the health of their patients.
> Investigation has established that members of this terrorist group, taking advantage of their status as physicians and abusing the trust of their patients, heinously undermined the health of the latter, deliberately ignored the data of objective examinations, made incorrect diagnoses which did not correspond to the nature of the ailments, and thus brought about the death of their charges by incorrect treatment.
> The criminals have admitted that they diagnosed incorrectly the illness of Comrade A. A. Zhdanov, concealing the myocardial infarction he had suffered and, by prescribing a regimen contraindicated in such a severe illness, caused the death of Comrade A. A. Zhdanov. The investigation estab-

lished that the criminals also cut short the life of Comrade A. S. Shcherbakov, by prescribing powerful drugs, recommending a detrimental regimen, and finally driving him to his death.

The criminal doctors concentrated their insidious activities on leading military men, trying to incapacitate them and so weaken the defense potential of the country. They tried to undermine the health of Marshal Vasilevsky, Marshal Govorov, Marshal Konev, Army General Shtemenko, Admiral Levchenko, and others. [Note that the mass shootings of major Soviet generals in 1937 did nothing to weaken the country's defense potential.] But the criminals were arrested before they succeeded in implementing their heinous designs.

It has been established that all these killer doctors, these monsters who trod underfoot the holy banner of science and defiled the honor of men of science, were in the pay of foreign intelligence services. Most members of the terrorist group (Vovsi, Kogan, Feldman, Grinstein, Etinger, and others) were connected with the international Jewish bourgeois nationalist organization Joint, which was set up by the American intelligence service allegedly for the purpose of rendering international aid to Jews in other countries. In actual fact, under the guidance of the CIA, this organization has been conducting espionage, terrorist, and other subversive activities in many countries, including the Soviet Union. Vovsi admitted to the investigators that via Dr. Shchimeliovich, living in Moscow, and the notorious Jewish bourgeois nationalist Mikhoels, Joint had directed him "to destroy leading statesmen of the USSR." It has been proved that other participants in the terrorist group (Vinogradov, Kogan, Yegorov) are long-standing agents of the British intelligence service.

The investigation will be concluded soon.

The news was absolutely mind-boggling, especially for those who knew the people mentioned in the Tass statement. They were all peace-loving, humane scientists and doctors, devoted to medicine heart and soul. Most of them were very far from

75

politics. I knew all of them well, for decades, as friends. Only a person whose faculties had been completely stupefied by the preceding show trials, beginning with the Shakhti case and the trial of the Prompartia (Industrial Party), could give credence to such allegations. This incredulity was best expressed by a BBC commentator, who said that any Englishman, upon hearing over the radio that King George had died not of old age but had been murdered by his physician, would have cried in horror: "A maniac must be at large in the BBC studio!"

Scant information penetrated our country concerning the reaction of foreign statesmen to this announcement and public opinion abroad (all channels of such information had been cut off). But even the little that reached the ears of Soviet citizens revealed active opposition. Attempts were made to influence the common sense of the Soviet leadership, or to awaken it. American President Dwight Eisenhower, one of the most popular figures in the postwar world, declared over the radio that he had issued instructions to make a thorough check into any connections that might have existed between the physicians arrested in the Soviet Union and American intelligence bodies, and he gave his word of honor that those organizations had never even heard the names of these "American spies" and had never been in touch with them or given them any assignments. Winston Churchill and other British statesmen also issued resolute denials of any contact between the British intelligence service and the people arrested in the USSR. Israel made strenuous efforts to clear Soviet Jews from the bloody imputations, which eclipsed even the Beilis case. (This was a trial held in Kiev in 1913 of a Jewish shop assistant Beilis, accused of murdering a Christian child for ritualistic purposes. The case was inspired by the Black Hundreds, and a wide wave of protest swept the country. Despite pressure from the tsarist government, the jury acquitted Beilis.) Indeed, the Doctors' Plot was designated "the Beilis case of the atomic age." The International Association of Democratic Lawyers, which had previously been actively pro-Soviet, demanded that its representatives be allowed to attend the trial of the killer doctors. The demand was rejected. Many other well-known intellectuals abroad, formerly friends of the Soviet Union, also expressed disbelief and criticism, and there is no doubt that the Doctors' Plot opened the eyes of many people to the true nature of Stalin's regime. Previously Stalin had managed to throw dust into the eyes of even such an astute author ("a wise old bird," in his own description) as Leon Feuchtwanger, who visited the Soviet Union in the fateful year 1937 and carried away the most delightful impressions of the person of Stalin, which he described in his book *Moscow, 1937*. Idealists, blinded by the legend about Stalin and the paradise he had created in Russia, could only be disenchanted by such an outrage as the Doctors' Plot.

Those who cooked up the script, "The Doctors' Plot, or the Scum of the Earth," had no knowledge of the principles of Greek tragedy. But instinct prompted them that light must be juxtaposed to darkness in this cock-and-bull story. The darkness was represented by a collection of white-smocked monsters bearing academic degrees and occupying high posts. The antipode, to equal them in luminosity, had to be on the level of the Mother of God or, at least, Joan of Arc. And such a luminary was found. This was one Lydia Timashuk, a rank-and-file doctor at the Kremlin Hospital, who worked in the cardiogram room. The luminary was also a secret agent of the MGB. Such agents were recruited in every establishment to report on anything untoward about employees, and, when facts were lacking, they invented them. Perhaps on her own initiative, but most probably on instructions from above, this Joan of Arc discovered intentional distortions in medical conclusions made by major medical experts who served as consultants in the hospital. She exposed their criminal designs and thus opened the eyes of security bodies to the existence of the infamous conspiracy.

The Soviet press went into raptures about the perspicacity and courage of this paragon of virtue. Poems were dedicated to her, she was styled "a great daughter of the Russian people," and near-religious veneration was accorded her. She was specifically compared to Joan of Arc. On January 20, 1953, the country's highest award, the Order of Lenin, was conferred on her for helping to unmask the killer doctors.

Not surprisingly, most people, blinded as they were by Stalin's stupefying propaganda, took the Tass statement about the killer doctors on faith. They were inured to staggering revelations, but this new one outshone by far all the previous concoctions. Not everyone had the sense to see in this yet another of Krylenko's fairy tales. Before he himself fell in a Stalinist purge, Nikolai Krylenko, a prominent figure in the party in the early years of the revolution, acted as prosecutor-general at a number of show trials of the 1930s, which handed out death sentences to many innocent people, including major statesmen and party workers.

So the statement of January 13, 1953, was accepted by many, including some medical personnel, as the truth. The reaction of the man in the street was twofold: hatred for "the scum of the earth" and the loss of faith in anyone wearing a doctor's white coat. Every physician was regarded as a potential murderer. I shall never forget the face of my laboratory assistant, distorted with fury and hatred, as she hissed through clenched teeth: "Damn intellectuals, they all deserve to be cudgeled." I have no doubt that if a cudgel had actually been placed in the hands of this woman, who if not terribly kind was not really bloodthirsty, she would not have hesitated to whack me on the head with it. Meetings were held at all factories and offices, some organized, some spontaneous, and almost all openly anti-semitic. Speakers would vehemently demand that the criminals should be put to a terrible death. Many went so far as to offer their services in carrying out the actual executions. Some offers were made by representatives of the medical profession, physicians and even professors, either because they were blind to reason or because they were trying to prove their own innocence and to disassociate themselves from their criminal colleagues. Passions ran high, fanned by the press, which staged an orgy of frenetic condemnation.

The stream of abuse in the newspapers had a distinct anti-semitic tone, set by the central official press. In its editorial published on January 13, which was obviously prepared before the official statement was released, *Izvestiya* stated:

> The actions of these monsters were masterminded by foreign intelligence services. Most of them have sold themselves, body and soul, to a branch of American intelligence, the international Jewish bourgeois nationalist organization Joint . . . The disgusting face of this foul Zionist espionage organization has now been fully exposed. It has been established that professional spies and assassins from Joint used as their agents corrupt Jewish bourgeois nationalists who have been conducting, under the guidance of the CIA, extensive spying, terrorist, and other subversive activities in many countries, the Soviet Union included. It was from this international Jewish bourgeois-nationalist organization, the off-spring of the American secret service, that the monster Vovsi received his instructions to destroy the top people in the USSR. These instructions were passed on to him by a Moscow doctor, Shchimeliovich, and the notorious Jewish bourgeois-nationalist Mikhoels. Other members of the terrorist group (Vinogradov, M. Kogan, Yegorov) have been proven to be long-standing agents of the British intelligence service.

The article also reminded readers that Kuibyshev, Menzhinsky, and Gorky had been murdered by the doctors Levin and Pletnyov.

Two brothers, Boris and Mikhail Kogan, were named among the monsters. Yet Boris was alleged to be an American spy, and Mikhail was a British agent. Obviously spying was a family profession, and, had there been more Kogan brothers, more foreign intelligence services would have benefited from their assistance. There is an interesting detail that received no notice in the Tass statement: Mikhail Kogan had died of cancer (which required the amputation of an arm) several years before being recruited by British intelligence. So he had to do his spying in the netherworld, a fact that in no way put off the MGB investigators. They did not scorn devilry if it suited their purposes, as I was soon to learn.

The satirical magazine *Krokodil* made its own contribution to the anathemizing of the Jewish killer doctors, cartoons that would have done honor to the Black Hundred press of tsarist times, which nauseated even conservative intellectuals of pre-revolutionary days. Of the mass of frankly antisemitic articles, the rabid lampoons by Olga Chechetkina were the most repulsive, reminiscent of the rabble-rousing boulevard publications of the pogrom period of 1904–05. A foul impression was also left by the articles of Gusta Fučikova, the widow of Czechoslovakia's hero Julius Fučik. It is hard to reconcile the tender lines dedicated by Fučik to his beloved wife in his "Reporting with a Noose around My Neck," whom he portrays as a sensitive and noble woman, with the viciousness of her writings on the killer doctors. Could these coarse vituperations have been written (and not just signed under duress) by the gentle woman of Fučik's description? Or did Fučik idealize her while he was in prison?

The Jews who remained at large had to add their own bit to inciting nationwide anti-Jewish indignation. A letter to *Pravda* was concocted that branded the killer doctors, and prominent Jewish scientists, musicians, composers, actors, and military men were asked to sign it. The letter's contents, I was later told, were not conspicuously original and boiled down to the following: "Soviet power has given Jews broad opportunities to apply their abilities in all spheres, but the despised monsters have paid back our generous state with unspeakable perfidy. The undersigned hereby announce that they disassociate themselves from these fiends and demand that the direst punishment be meted out to them." Almost all who were approached signed the letter.

I will not mention the names; some of them (I have been told) are world-famous. They were victims of the times, just like the unfortunates they condemned with *Pravda*-inspired fervor. The composer Blanter said to me that, after he had signed the letter, he opened *Pravda* with trembling hands every morning, expecting to see the abominable document over his signature. But I feel duty-bound to name those who had the courage to refuse to sign the letter. They were the opera singer Mark Reisen, Colonel-General Yakov Kreiser, who commanded a cavalry corps of Cossacks during the war, the writer Ilya Ehrenburg, and the composer Isaac Dunayevsky. There was a misunderstanding of a somewhat comical nature with respect to the composer Reinhold Glier. When approached, he said that he was prepared to sign the letter, but he was not a Jew, for his father was a German and his mother a Ukrainian. After this explanation, the honor of signing the letter was withdrawn.

The document never saw the light of day. Either it was decided that "good Jews" were not required at the moment (in light of the repressions planned against the entire nationality in the near future), or perhaps the publication was delayed for some reason and lost its point after Stalin's death. But the very fact of the fabrication of such a letter adds color to the moral panorama of Stalin's era.

Moscow always set an example for the rest of the Soviet Union. So it did in the fabrication of the Doctors' Plot. In every big city and even in provincial towns, local murderers in white coats were rooted out. Only the MGB bodies have exact figures on how many people were arrested. The lists of doctors exonerated after Stalin's death, which were published in the newspapers on April 4, were far from complete. Of the people I personally knew to have been arrested, the lists omitted Vladimir Zelenin, Boris Zbarsky, Eliazar Gelstein, Ginda Bykhovskaya, Mark Sereisky, Joseph Feugel, Veniamin Nezlin,

Naum Vilk, my own name, and many others, not to mention their wives. It was apparently decided that the lists had to be abridged; otherwise it would have been easier to publish the names of those who had not been arrested. In a number of big cities, especially in the Ukraine, all Jewish professors who had escaped arrest were expelled from the medical schools (later most were reinstated).

There was one case that was close to our family. My wife's brother Grigory Epstein, a prominent specialist in traumas, was fired from the two posts he held in Leningrad: head of the traumatology department of Leningrad Institute of Advanced Training for Doctors, and department head at the Vreden Institute of Traumatology in Leningrad. Finding himself out of a job, he came to Moscow to the personnel board of the Ministry of Health to ask for an assignment. The personnel board manager, Trofimov, who received him, offered him the post of general practitioner in the Yakutsk Autonomous Republic, the kind of job that is usually given to recent graduates from medical school. To Epstein's query as to whether he, Trofimov, considered it expedient to disregard his scientific and professional knowledge and experience, and in view of his age (fifty-seven), the reply was blunt: "I can offer nothing else to such as you. I'd advise you to accept because very soon I may be unable even to offer you that much." This was a clear hint that more rigors were in store for Jews: pogroms and mass resettlement to the outer reaches of Siberia.

Someone told me the following story, vouching for its authenticity. The hero is a pediatrician, a professor from Kiev, who had been treating the children of a major political and party functionary of the Ukraine; he had in fact been their family doctor, greatly respected and liked by his young patients and their parents. After January 13, he was discharged from the polyclinic that looked after the health of top officials in the Ukraine. After a while, the mother of his erstwhile charges phoned him and asked him to see one of the children. The doctor was no longer entitled to do so, of which he informed her, but she insisted. So he came, examined the child, and wrote a prescription. To his surprise, the mother asked him not to leave yet. He wondered if she intended to pay him as for a private consultation. A few minutes later, he was invited to the study where he found the child's father, who was there especially to see him. Without explaining anything, he asked the professor if he could see a way to leave Kiev at once and settle in some out-of-the-way town. It was a friendly warning. The professor never followed the advice of this good man, who risked quite a lot should the conversation become known to anyone outside the family. The unexpected happy finale of the doctors' case made flight unnecessary.

The public mood after the government announcement about the killer doctors and the hidden mechanism of the affair could be likened to the so-called cholera rebellions of an earlier age. This name was given to rebellions that flared up in the Russian countryside in the nineteenth century during severe epidemics of cholera. These explosions of fury, which had accumulated over decades of poverty and starvation, were often directed against doctors and nurses who battled the terrible disease. The ignorant and superstitious peasants blamed the doctors for spreading the disease, and many fell victim to this misguided anger. The rebels often went on to attack their age-old oppressors—government officials and landowners—and the rebellions acquired such scope that special punitive measures had to be taken. "God forbid that we see a Russian rebellion, senseless and merciless," wrote Alexander Pushkin of Pugachev's bloody peasant revolt.

The Doctors' Plot of 1953 was yet another such rebellion, but transplanted to the twentieth century and Stalin's empire. The only difference was that the cholera rebellions were a spontaneous expression of popular rage, while the Soviet rebellion was carefully engineered and the fury of the people was purposefully fanned. As in the nineteenth century, its first and main objects were physicians, to whom terrible crimes were imputed. As in the nineteenth century, the anger of the misguided people spread from doctors to intellectuals in general (recall the words of my laboratory assistant—"Damn intellectuals, they all deserve to be cudgeled").

The other reaction to the Tass announcement was a horror of all medicine. Every doctor was regarded as a saboteur, and to seek any medical aid at all was considered dangerous. Rumors were spread about alleged deterioration of health after doctors' prescribed treatments. As a matter of fact, this is feasible, for no treatment can guarantee immediate improvement. On some occasions symptoms may mount until the climax in the course of the illness is reached. But at that time such facts were regarded by the frightened man in the street as evidence of criminal intent.

"True" stories were spread about a patient's death immediately after a doctor's visit. The doctor in question was allegedly arrested and shot at once. Newborn infants, it was said, were being killed by doctors in maternity wards. Clinic attendance fell sharply and pharmacies were empty—all as a result of rumors about cases when a sharp turn for the worse occurred after some seemingly innocuous medicine was taken. I remember the following episode. A young mother came to the Tarasevich Institute, where I was still working, and brought an empty penicillin phial. Her baby was ill with pneumonia and, according to her, its condition had sharply deteriorated after an injection of penicillin. An allergic reaction to antibiotics is not infrequent. Yet she demanded that the phial be analyzed for poison. She announced that she would not give any more medicine to her baby. When I said that she was endangering the child's life, she declared with frenzied determination that she would prefer her baby to die of pneumonia rather than poison.

The threat of dire consequences dogged all doctors, especially Jews, if patient or family imagined that there was something wrong in the treatment. Some people actually threatened to prosecute. I myself saw such a "solicitous" husband in the admission ward of the First Gradskaya Hospital. Pad and pen in hand, he demanded to know and wrote down the name of the doctor who admitted his wife, the ward where she was to be placed, the head doctor of the department, and the ward doctor. He made no bones about his intention to take the doctors to court should anything go wrong with his wife. Such an attitude, far from enhancing a doctor's sense of responsibility, served only to breed anxiety and fear among medical personnel. Doctors tended to be overcautious and to think of their own safety rather than of the patient's health. The physical and moral harm done by the Doctors' Plot has not yet been fully assessed.

– 6 –

My Arrest

I HAD the distinct feeling of a rope tightening around my neck. The meaning of some events became clear to me only after my arrest. One such event was a summons to the district military registration office in December 1952, a few weeks before my arrest. A similar summons had been received by my close friend Eliazar Gelstein. By then he had been fired from the Second Medical Institute, where he had headed the therapy department. He was simply pensioned off, since he had had two heart attacks (as a consequence of the hounding that preceded his discharge) and had developed a chronic cardiac aneurysm; he was totally disabled. What he told me about his visit to the military registration office was most perplexing. The purpose of the summons, he was told, was to receive a physical exam as a war veteran. He informed the medical commission about the state of his health, showing them the cardiograms testifying to the poor condition of his heart. As a matter of fact, his condition was obvious even without the cardiograms. To his amazement, the medical commission declared him fit for military service both in peacetime and in war, that is, it gave him a clean bill of health. He told the commission members that they were committing a grave medical error. Then they called in the head of the registration office to arbitrate. A colonel entered and, looking at poor Gelstein, pronounced: "He looks fit enough for military service." All this was baffling. What perplexed Gelstein most was that the medical commission deferred to the colonel's opinion, formed by a casual glance. I have no doubt that the man was not the head of that registration office but an MGB colonel.

Several days later, I was summoned there too. The young captain who received me said that the army did not need pathologists just then and did not foresee such a need in the near future, that they intended to discharge me from the reserves, but that it was necessary first to have a physical. Before demobilization, in the spring of 1945, because of hypertension and an injury, I had been declared only partially fit for military service. I wondered what the point of a physical was now if it had already been decided to strike my name from the register, but figured it was just another army formality. The medical commission, which consisted of several persons, spoke to me quite amiably, discussed hypertension as such without examining me at all, and let me go under the impression that this had been a technicality requiring no special medical competence or even a rudimentary sort of investigation. Imagine my surprise when, the next day, I found on my registration card not the mark of discharge from military service but a stamp certifying my fitness for service both in peacetime and in war. I could not understand it. Only later, after the events of 1953, did I realize that the procedure had a purpose: if I was declared fit for military service, then I was also fit for prison. The same applied to Gelstein.

On January 14, the day after the publication of the Tass statement, the head doctor of the First Gradskaya Hospital informed me that I had been relieved of my post as pathologist at the hospital, since my main post was at the Tarasevich Institute. This was obviously a pretext, since most heads of hospital departments who held the academic rank of professor had their main jobs in the establishments where they held professorial posts. The head doctor (Lev Chernyshev) advised me in strong terms not to dispute the decision, hinting that it had been approved by the top people or perhaps even came directly from them. I had no intention of complaining anyway, since I knew why I was being sacked. My subordinates, I discovered when I returned to my office, already knew about the expulsion, and the atmosphere was funereal. Nobody said much, but I was shocked to see my old laboratory worker Yefim Ryzhkov, who had been with me for nearly thirty years, suddenly burst into tears. Apparently he realized what was in store for me. I handed over my department to Nadezhda Arkhangelskaya, who was to take up my post.

Two days after my discharge, I had a telephone call from the hospital. I was invited to a meeting in connection with the Tass statement about the killer doctors. This statement mentioned, as an active saboteur, Yakov Etinger. The clinic he had headed before his discharge was part of the First Gradskaya Hospital. So was the clinic of Vladimir Vinogradov, before the war. Since I was no longer employed at the hospital, I could refuse to go. But precisely because the matter concerned Etinger, who was my good friend, I decided to attend. I don't remember exactly what was said by the speakers—much the same, I suppose, that was said at other such meetings at the time. Particularly rabid was Zolotova-Kostomarova, Etinger's former assistant and his most remorseless and frenzied persecutor, who stepped into his shoes after the expulsion but did not manage to hold the post for long.

In my speech I said that I had been shattered by the statement about the monstrous crimes performed by prominent people in the medical profession, including Yakov Etinger. I had known many of these people for a long time and was close to quite a few. Many of those present also knew them and knew what authority and respect they enjoyed. Like many others, of course, I could never imagine that these people were capable of such heinous deeds. Even now, I said, I could not believe that the impression I had formed over many years of acquaintance was the result of a masquerade. I could not side with those who said that they had long suspected Etinger of being a traitor and a potential murderer, for if I had I would have acted against what was demanded by my civic duty and my conscience.

This was my last contact with the First Gradskaya Hospital before my arrest. I crossed its threshold again only five years later—and in entirely different circumstances.

The grim events were marching on. Shells burst ever closer, and the terrible feeling mounted that one of them would soon make a direct hit. The premonition was strengthened by the arrest, on January 25, of Vladimir Zelenin, a prominent internist, my own and my wife's teacher and a family friend. At that time my wife was in Toropets where our daughter Naomi was working. When I told my wife over the telephone that Zelenin had been arrested, she left Toropets at once. By some unfathomable psychological mechanism, she ascribed a fateful importance to this particular piece of news, although information about arrests had been coming in a steady stream.

During our life together, Sophia and I had spoken about the possibility of my arrest on many occasions. Why should I be spared when so many people we knew, friends and relatives, honest and devoted Soviet citizens, had been taken from us? I had committed a few acts that were imprudent by the notions of those times. So my wife always kept ready for me a set of the basic necessities—a change of underwear, handkerchiefs, soap—things I might need "there." Now that arrest seemed imminent, we again discussed the stand I was to take at interrogations. Sophia was convinced that the firing squad unavoidably awaited those who had not been able to withstand torture, of which blood-curdling rumors were floating about, and had signed admissions of guilt. So she implored me to be steadfast, to mobilize all my courage, to bear all tortures, and not to sign anything. I always remembered this plea of hers; it sustained me in prison, at the most difficult moments. We heard that the security forces had broadened the notion of crime to the point of absurdity, and the most innocuous action performed every day by a normal person could be represented as a monstrous crime against party and state. My personal experience confirmed this, and my investigators initiated me into some of the principles of Soviet criminology formulated by that man of infamous memory, Vyshinsky. Even children knew that any trifle could be classified as a political crime. Evidence of this is the following joke my daughter Natasha brought home from school: A bear, a wolf, and a cockerel are confined in a prison cell and tell each other about the crimes they are guilty of. The bear says: "I killed a cow." The wolf says: "I killed a sheep." And the cockerel says: "My crime is political—I pecked a Young Pioneer on the ass."

Then came the fateful day of February 3. I was sitting as an official opponent at a thesis defense at the Medical Academy. After this I went to the Scientists' Club to get some foreign medical journals for myself and Gelstein, who was too ill to travel about the city. In the evening I called to tell him what journals I had collected, but nobody answered. That seemed very strange, since I knew that Gelstein was seriously ill and that, moreover, his wife, Ginda Bykhovskaya, a well-known neurologist, should also be at home. Finally, at ten in the evening, I got through. Their maid told me in a panicky voice that the Gelsteins had just been arrested and taken away after a search that had lasted for twenty-four hours. This shell had burst right next to me, and I had no doubt that the next one would get me. That evening we were to go to a party at the Moshkovskys', in our apartment building. I took my savings with me and asked the Moshkovskys to keep the money for my family after my arrest. It was a dismal evening. All of us thought, even though we did not put it into words, that we were parting forever. But each man secretly hoped that fate would spare him and his family. I was the only one without a grain of hope, though I am optimistic by nature.

When we got back to our entrance hall, it was well after midnight. We were surprised to see that the elevator attendant, who usually left at twelve and locked the elevator, was still there. Beside her stood a man in civilian clothes who looked like a thug. As we were going up in the elevator, I suggested to my wife that he must be an MGB man. Sophia, who often had occasion to see "that kind" on the landings of our stairwell, as they watched somebody in the yard without the slightest attempt at disguise, said he didn't have the right look. The man was in fact a member of the group that had come to arrest me. His function was either to watch the elevator attendant, lest she get away and warn me about the nocturnal visitors, or to grab me if I attempted to escape. When I unlocked my door and entered the hall, I realized what was afoot. In the hall, to the right of the door, stood a young man in the regulation plain clothes of the MGB (a blue coat with a gray astrakhan collar and an astrakhan hat). He greeted me with an insolent grin. The door to the brightly lit dining room stood open, and I saw, or rather sensed, the presence of many people there. I was prepared for all this psychologically, so much so that I said to the man in the hall, "Oh, hi!" This was not bravado, still less was it a host's greeting. What my exclamation implied was, "At last!" In the same way, death relieves a person of the terror of expecting it.

In response to my greeting, my guest began searching my pockets, asking the standard question: "Any firearms?" When I entered the dining room, I found a large group of people: two or three young MGB men in uniform, an elderly colonel, the building's caretaker, who must have been brought in to act as a witness, and our young maid. Both women looked frightened and depressed. The colonel showed me the warrant for my arrest and for the search of the apartment, which I did not bother to read, since neither its wording nor the person who signed it had the slightest significance for me. I just noted that it was issued the day before, February 2. As I later learned, the order for Gelstein's arrest was issued the same day, but the MGB force must have been overtaxed with work, and so I was left at large for a day longer.

I don't remember all the details of the procedure that followed, nor are they of much interest. The colonel spoke to my wife in a calm and even solicitous tone, advising her what things I should take along "for the road," adding that no food was allowed. I took leave of my wife, carrying away in my memory the earnest injunction, "Courage!" which she uttered at the very last moment, and, bundle in hand, I set out into the unknown escorted by the colonel. As we walked down the stairs, the colonel said, "If you meet a neighbor, say you are going on a business trip." I did not reply to this naive piece of advice: Soviet people knew only too well what kind of trip awaited those who left their homes in the middle of the night, accompanied by an MGB colonel. Downstairs, by the elevator cage, I saw neither the attendant nor the thug. I got into a car that was standing by the curb. On the way I asked only one question, more of myself rather than of the colonel: "What can I be accused of?" The colonel answered in comforting tones, "Perhaps they need you as a witness." This surprised me so greatly that I said: "Do they arrest witnesses?" He answered: "Sometimes it is necessary to have them isolated." The rest of the journey across nocturnal Moscow passed in oppressive silence, until the heavy gates of the huge building in Lubyanka Street swung open before our car (on the Sretenka Street side) and the car drove into the yard. Such was the beginning of a new stage in my life, whose end was obscured in impenetrable darkness—perhaps in the netherworld.

I recall everything that followed as a horrible dream with blackouts (the proceedings probably also had that quality at the time). My memory has retained only individual occurrences, and, try as I might, I cannot recall the sequence of events of that first night. I only remember that, in the beginning, I failed fully to comprehend the grim implications of what was happening and was even feeling an objective researcher's curiosity about what was in store for me. As I mentioned, along the way to the Lubyanka, I racked my brains about what charges could have been brought against me. I did not have to wait long to be enlightened. After a short stay in a tiny cell, I was led into a room where a young man wearing the uniform of an MGB captain was sitting behind a desk with a stony and contemptuously severe expression on his face. As I entered the room I said, out of force of habit, "Good evening." This kind of automatic courtesy never deserts me, not even when I am driving a car and hear obscenities from another driver on account of some error I have committed. To such abuse I invariably respond with "I'm sorry."

The captain informed me that he was an investigator. During our subsequent meetings I learned the name of "Citizen Investigator," as I was to address him: it was Roman Yevgenievich Odlyanitsky. He was about thirty, with a narrow face and a smattering of education. There was also something sly about him. He responded to my greeting with a barely perceptible nod and a grunt. This was probably as much as a man under arrest was entitled to. With no introduction he announced to me: "You have been arrested as a Jewish bourgeois nationalist, an enemy of the Soviet people. So tell me about your crimes." This declaration quite satisfied my curiosity, and I even felt a kind of relief—not because my curiosity was satisfied but because I imagined I would have no trouble disproving such absurd charges. I shall say in advance that I was wrong, for I had no idea what interpretation the MGB gave to the concept of "Jewish bourgeois nationalism." I could have cited countless examples of my patriotism and love for Russia, which sentiments helped me to bear the many insults and trials that fell to my lot as a Jew. My sense of dignity never permitted me to bring forth testimony of my love for my country—not in any circumstances. Nor did I try to prove it in prison.

So I said to the investigator with sincere conviction that I had never been a Jewish bourgeois nationalist and had never committed any crimes against the Soviet people. The investigator then repeated the formulaic charge and demanded that I should stop denying my guilt and give an account of my crimes. I asked him what crimes exactly were imputed to me, for if I were told in concrete terms I should be able to say if I had committed them or not. To this he quickly replied: "That won't do! You shall tell me everything of your own accord." Subsequently I realized that a person being interrogated by the MGB was supposed to invent his own crimes, for these upholders of justice did not want to be bothered with the task. These exchanges continued for about an hour. Toward the end the investigator threatened me: "You'd better come clean, then you'll stay here. This is no health resort, to be sure, but the conditions are quite decent. If you continue to deny everything, I'll report to my superiors, and you will be put on a special regime." This threat, the meaning of which was not at all clear to me, had no effect. The investigator started writing something and went on with it for quite a long time. Then he suggested that I sign the examination record, which he called "the protocol." This was my first acquaintance with his peculiar style. The protocol consisted of questions and answers, and I have retained the memory of the general style and content of the initial ones:

> *Question.* You, Rapoport, have been arrested as a Jewish bourgeois nationalist, an enemy of the people. Tell me about your crimes.
> *Answer.* I have committed no crimes.
> *Question.* This is a hipocritical lie. ["Hipocritical" is his spelling, not mine; even in that atmosphere, I retained an editor's habit of noticing spelling mistakes.]
> *Answer.* There is no hipocrisy here.
> *Question.* Stop quibbling and tell me about your vile deeds.
> *Answer.* I have never committed any vile deeds.
> *Question.* You will not evade responsibility for your crimes, Rapoport.
> *Answer.* I have committed no crimes . . .

This stupid quiz, under the heading "Protocol of the Interrogation," took up a page. At the bottom, the interrogator and I signed, and the man left the room.

94

In his place appeared someone who looked like a soldier. He put a dirty napkin on my shoulders, and I was initiated into the brotherhood of jailbirds—my hair was shaved off. After this I was forced to take a shower (they were quite solicitous about prisoners' hygiene at the MGB). After the shower I was made to stand before a lukewarm radiator and told, "Dry off!" I did my best to do so, relying more on my body warmth than on the radiator. As I was drying off, my trousers, coat, and shoes were carefully examined. The buttons, on which some letters denoting the manufacturer were embossed, were cut off, and thereafter my trousers stayed in place only out of their touching devotion to me, supported by a single illiterate button. It is impossible to fathom the secret meaning behind the deprivation of the trousers and coat of their buttons, unless one is to believe that anti-Soviet propaganda had been stamped there by some subversive firm. The laces were taken out of my shoes—obviously to prevent me from hanging myself.

Shaved, washed, dried, and shorn of buttons, I was packed into a Black Raven and posted deeper into the unknown. The design of these vehicles has been described many times in our literature (in the west they are called Black Marias). But I shall give yet another description of this conveyance for the uninitiated, especially since in the intervening decades technology has made big strides, and other means are probably used for transporting prisoners today. My Black Raven was an ordinary van, like those used to carry foodstuffs. A narrow aisle ran down the middle, dividing it into two parts, each of which was subdivided into several small cubicles. They were just big enough to accommodate a person of average corpulence. At the back of each cubicle was a bench for enforced sitting with your knees pushing against the cubicle's door. There was an eyehole in that door, through which the guard could take a look at the passenger's face, lit by a weak electric bulb. In the back there was a metal door, as on any van.

We started on our way. It was a long trip. We crossed railroad tracks and stood a long time at a crossing on a turnpike, for I heard the noise of a passing train. Then there was a stop, for at least half an hour, if my sense of time had not gone haywire in that hermetically sealed apparatus. The guards had apparently left on some business of their own (probably to have a mug of beer, for it was late morning by then). Upon their return they inquired with touching solicitude: "Hey you, aren't frozen stiff, are you?" and, satisfied by my answer (my pride prevented me from admitting that I was indeed frozen stiff), climbed into the van. It was afternoon when we finally drove into some kind of yard (I guessed this from the sound of gates being unlocked and then locked again) and, on emerging from my cosy compartment, I saw that I was obviously in a prison.

I was taken into a room on the ground floor where a woman of about thirty with a pleasant, kindly face, wearing a doctor's white coat, told me to undress. I imagined that I was to undergo a conventional medical checkup, for which purpose I took off my coat and shirt, and I was surprised and embarrassed (having not yet lost my sense of manhood) by her suggestion that I should strip naked. But there was no way to refuse, especially since a guard was present. The nice-looking doctor examined all my orifices (ears, nose, throat), ending with the anus, into which she inserted a finger as far as it would go (it was a good thing the examination did not proceed in the reverse order). Doing the latter, she suddenly pronounced, "No piles," as if pleasantly surprised at the absence of piles in an elderly Jewish professor. I could not resist the temptation to ask, "Don't they shoot people who have no piles?" She obviously failed to appreciate my sense of humor (apparently humor was a rare guest in this establishment) and gave me a surprised and, as I imagined, interested glance. Perhaps she knew me, as many physicians did, as a lecturer and speaker at scientific conferences. It was only recently that I stumbled across the reason for such a heightened interest in the orifices of my body: I might have had an ampule of poison on my person. Before this I used to tell my friends jokingly that she must have been looking for an atomic bomb or a quick-firing gun.

96

What was happening at home in the meantime? My wife told me about it when I returned from the "house of the dead." (I refer to this return as exhumation, which was not far from the truth.) The MGB people who remained behind started searching the apartment. Later they also searched my dacha, where they went accompanied by my wife. The search was very thorough; each nook and corner was examined for compromising evidence. I found the aftermath of this search when I came back, and the two rooms they had sealed were opened. On the floor lay a heap of assorted things: books, collections of medical slides, my research papers. They went through the lot with a fine-toothed comb but for a long time failed to hit on anything clearly counterrevolutionary that testified to my membership in a terrorist organization. At any rate, they kept ringing up somebody to report the scarcity of finds. And suddenly there was general excitement: they had found poison! It was a square box with atropine ampules bearing the warning sign—the skull and crossbones—that is put on any dangerous medicine. I kept atropine in my medicine chest for an emergency—a possible attack of the coronary insufficiency I was subject to. The find was immediately telephoned to "Comrade General" at the MGB. One might have thought they had discovered bombs, machine guns, or the other paraphernalia of a terrorist. To be sure, though, poison is the weapon of a killer doctor, who murders his trusting patients with poison and not a gun. The sensation spread all over the building: poison had been found in Rapoport's apartment! (There were also "reliable reports" that I took pus from the terminally ill and used it to infect healthy people.) The terrible box was sealed, and I later saw it in my investigator's hands. By then the seal had been broken and one ampule was missing—it had obviously been sent for analysis, which must have established the nature of its contents. Nevertheless, the investigator asked me: "Why did you keep poison in your house? Did you intend to kill yourself when being arrested?" He seemed to imagine that I was going to follow the example of Hitler, Himmler, and other Nazis, being, as he saw it, their heir and adherent. To this I replied that I had no reason to kill myself and had made no preparations for suicide. Besides, the investigator must be aware of the purpose of this medicine. There was no further mention of poison during the investigation: either the find was considered a flop, or other questions overshadowed it; it is also possible that they were saving it for the detailed conclusion to my terrorist confession.

Other things classified as compromising and taken away were a hunting knife in a leather sheath and a small Nazi flag with a swastika. The knife (so blunt, incidentally, that it could not even cut bread) was a present from the head of a hospital at the Karelian front, where I served in the war. It had been made by an orderly who was a master craftsman. Such knives were in the possession of almost all military personnel in Finland, a kind of local souvenir. My knife could never have been used as a weapon, blunt as it was, and even the sheath did not lend it the sinister appearance of a pigsticker. As for the flag, I had picked it up from a desk at the German headquarters in Riga recently evacuated by the Nazis. I kept it as a kind of trophy, but, to preclude any possible accusation of sympathy with the Nazis, I wrote on it in ink the date and place I had obtained it: Riga, October 13, 1944 (the day the city was liberated). Nevertheless, the investigator asked me, "Where did you get the German swastika? I could understand your keeping an American stars and stripes, but a Nazi swastika—it's too much for a Jew!" I then drew his attention to the inscription on the flag, which explained its origin. This matter, too, was never raised again, but the two objects might eventually have been accepted as evidence of guilt, if the investigation ever reached its conclusion.

There were countless examples of the use made by the MGB of the most absurd evidence to prove a person's criminal activities or intent. This came to light during the study of cases for the purpose of rehabilitating those incarcerated innocently. Surely a blunt knife and atropine ampules were no less convincing evidence than the bent barrel of a machine gun from a

German plane shot down near Moscow. Yet this same barrel, which some boys found near the spot where the plane exploded, was the chief piece of material evidence of a conspiracy on the part of a group of young people, "uncovered" by the MGB in 1943. These youngsters were the children of people shot or imprisoned in the 1930s, and they were alleged to have formed an organization to avenge their parents. (I was told about this case by the son of our family friend Zinaida Kieselstein, who was sentenced to a term in a concentration camp, survived it, and returned.)

This bent machine-gun barrel, found in the apartment of one boy during a search, was to figure as irrefutable proof of guilt. One of the youths admitted under torture that they intended to machine-gun Stalin's car as it drove along Arbat Street (his usual route) from the window of the room in which one of the female members of the group lived. Neither this absurd material evidence, nor the fact that the window in question faced an inner yard and not the street, prevented the judges from meting out harsh sentences. So I cannot be sure that the blunt knife and the swastika might not have figured prominently in my own case, although the investigator did not seem to attach much importance to them at the time.

The search at my home continued for almost forty-eight hours; many letters and documents were taken away. Of our four rooms, two were sealed off; my wife and younger daughter Natasha, a schoolgirl, lived in the other two. Some of our possessions, which were apparently subject to confiscation after I was sentenced, were moved to the rooms that were sealed off, and some were left for my family to use, though my wife was made to sign for them. The most aggressive of the men who conducted the search was the one who had searched my person for weapons; the others, younger MGB men, behaved more peaceably and even expostulated with the older man over some points. For instance, he demanded that the upright piano should be moved to the rooms that were to be sealed, but the others objected, pointing out that my daughter used it. On discovering my collection of tsarist banknotes, he wanted to add it to the compromising material, arguing that the money had been paid to me for my subversive activities by the American intelligence service, but the others reasoned that it was obviously "Natasha's collection." This I regard as confirmation of the belief I share with the poet Sasha Chorny, that "not only curs live on this earth of ours."

Among the materials taken away were the letters I exchanged with my wife when one of us was away on business or holiday. My wife saved all my letters throughout the many years of our marriage. Like many members of my profession, I have an illegible hand and it takes some getting used to. All my correspondents tell me that, at each new reading, they discover something new in my letters. My investigator once asked me to read a passage from one of my letters that he could not decipher. I said I was not always able to read my own writing and that the job of deciphering all my letters would last the time it would take three MGB lieutenants to retire with the rank of general. All my correspondence was eventually returned to me and, looking through it, I found a letter my wife wrote to me when I was taking a holiday in the Crimea in 1938. It could have been used as a conclusive piece of evidence against me, proof of my close connection with the criminal organization of Jewish terrorists. My wife wrote that Miron Vovsi had been looking for me. His clinic was part of the Botkin Hospital, where Shchimeliovich, named as the ringleader in the Tass statement, was chief physician. By the time of my arrest, Shchimeliovich had already been executed (on August 12, 1952) along with the other twenty-four members of the Jewish Anti-Fascist Committee. After January 13, 1953, the names of Vovsi and Shchimeliovich were bugbears, and any connections with them were suspect. Suffice it to say that the dacha cooperative (to which I also belonged) called a meeting of the board to consider the expulsion of a man who had rented his country house to Vovsi.

It must be noted that this cooperative was long subject to pillaging practices pursued by people with academic titles who were also members of the Communist Party. Many of our cooperative members had fallen victim to the epidemic of arrests in 1937–38. As soon as the news reached the board, they would expel the arrested man, throw his family out on their ear, and hand the dacha over to their own friends and relatives, who paid only the "balance due" (usually only a small portion of the actual value). On some occasions even this payment was not demanded, and the new owner became entitled to whatever money the rightful owner had already paid to cover expenses. This was outright robbery of unfortunate people, camouflaged by high-sounding phrases about disassociation from an "enemy of the people." As a matter of fact, the operation was often carried out before the sentence involving confiscation of property was actually passed. At that terrible time, an arrest was in itself a sentence, and the shattered family, if any members were left at large, never dared to protest or sue the cooperative, since no legal or other Soviet establishment would have undertaken to protect them. The same happened now in my case. As soon as I was arrested (information about the arrest immediately reached the board members, since my dacha was also subjected to a search). I was expelled from the cooperative , and my house was handed over to an MGB colonel who arrived with his wife to look over the gift. Unluckily for the colonel, he did not have enough time actually to take possession of the dacha. Had the documents been made out in his name, I would never have been able to get it back.

To return to my wife's letter. She wrote that Vovsi and Shchimeliovich wanted me to leave the First Gradskaya Hospital and take the post of head of the pathology department at the Botkin Hospital. There can be no doubt that the MGB investigators could have given this idea a sinister interpretation: so the terrorists had already tried to recruit me in 1938 to cover up their crimes! This letter would surely have led me to death row. (Vovsi's and Shchimeliovich's plan was never realized because it met with opposition from the management of the hospital and institute where I was then employed.)

I have already described the reaction of the outside world to the arrest of the killer doctors. How did the microworld, my own environment, react to my arrest? The general feeling for my wife was one of sympathy and commiseration, silent, as a rule, but clearly felt. Occasionally somebody would dare whisper an inquiry about me, and the answer was always, "I have not heard from him."

Some people were more forthright in expressing their sympathy, and of these I owe the greatest debt of gratitude to the Beklemishevs. They were our building neighbors on the floor below. The head of the family, Vladimir Nikolaevich Beklemishev, was a prominent entomologist, a member of the Academy of Medical Sciences. He represented that type of Russian intellectual, selfless and pure-minded, whom we know from the works of Turgenev, Tolstoy, Chekhov, and other writers of the prerevolutionary era, a type that has sadly disappeared. Even his external appearance was in accord with our idea of the intellectual: he was tall, spare, straight as a rod, and had a goatee. His amazing breadth of interests embraced history, literature, and ethnography, a knowledge acquired from literary sources that he was able to read in modern European languages and also in Greek and Latin. Also he was a religious man, though he did not attend church, and in his bedroom study hung an icon of Christ. On meeting him, one was left with the impression of a nobility of spirit radiating from his kindly, somewhat innocent eyes, although he was by no means a simple person. His wife, Nina Petrovna, was an ideal partner—a glowing, high-spirited, amiable woman, but with considerable worldly acumen.

Vladimir reacted to my arrest in a special way. On meeting my wife, he did not merely exchange the time of day with her, which was not done even by some of our closest friends, but he took off his hat and bowed to her from the waist. This bow was not merely an expression of sympathy, it was more like homage to a martyr. His wife Nina, for her part, visited my wife shortly after my arrest, at a time when the brand of "enemy of the people" surrounded my family with an impenetrable wall.

Even close friends did not come. Nina Petrovna offered money to my wife, but she refused. My wife also received great moral support—which she sorely needed in those grim days—from our close friends the Moshkovskys, both parents and children, the wonderful Guber family, and many others.

Aunt Xenia had been our children's nanny, and when they grew up and we moved into a new condominium building for medical personnel, we got her the job of elevator attendant, which was much easier than being a nanny, and she was given a little apartment of her own. She chided the MGB people who came to arrest me: "Shame on you, how can you arrest a man like that!" Even the investigator knew about her warm feelings for our family. He said to me once that, at any rate, my family had a devoted nanny to rely on. Aunt Xenia asked her priest whether the church allowed her to pray for a Jew. The priest said of course she could, and Aunt Xenia was firmly convinced that her prayers saved my life. Prayers for me were also said by an old friend of ours, an elderly Jewish woman, who supplemented her supplications to the Jewish God by a lengthy fast. So the Russian and Jewish gods joined efforts to rescue a godless atheist. As I learned later, many friends and acquaintances of mine who were not religious also turned to God, for there were no earthly powers they could appeal to.

As an example of very different moral principles, I can name another of our neighbors, Genokh Kogan, a Jew. His daughter was a classmate of my Natasha, and Natasha had often helped the girl with her lessons. After my arrest, Natasha decided to return some copybooks she had left at our place. The door was opened by the father. At the sight of my daughter, he bellowed: "How dare you come here, you dirty scum!" and gave Natasha such a shove in the chest that she nearly fell down the stairs. The copybooks scattered on the floor, and Natasha ran away, to remember that episode for the rest of her life.

The reaction of Natasha's classmates (she was fourteen at the time) was yet another proof that Stalin had not reduced all Soviet people to the condition of unthinking brutes. As a rule, when a student's parents were arrested, the Young Pioneer's red tie was symbolically taken from the child's neck at a solemn ceremony, and he or she was expelled from the organization. In 1937 I chanced to overhear a snatch of a conversation between two schoolboys, who were laughing over just such an occasion: "Grishka sure bawled when they tore the tie off his neck!" Many of Natasha's friends and classmates who lived in the neighboring houses knew about my arrest, but not one ever mentioned it at school. It was a spontaneous conspiracy of silence. This self-imposed pledge was broken only when I was released, and Natasha's classmates came to congratulate her.

One event that occurred several days before my arrest added spice to the situation. The teacher of history and geography at Natasha's school was an odd person, obviously somewhat unbalanced. She asked Natasha about the Constitution of the United States, and though Natasha spoke extensively and well, she gave her not an A but only a C. The other students, who were indignant at the injustice, asked the teacher why she had given Natasha a lower mark than she deserved. The teacher explained it as follows: "Didn't you notice how she spoke about America?" and she mimicked Natasha derisively: " 'It is such a wonderful country, life is so good there; I shall go there soon to visit my aunt!'" The teacher had invented this aunt in her accusatory zeal. Coming home, Natasha told us about the incident, and I decided not to let the accusation hang. Someone was bound to ascribe this admiration of the American way of life to the pupil's parents. So my wife and I went to see the principal together. She had happened to be present at the lesson, and so we asked her if she had any criticism to offer about Natasha's exposition. Not knowing what it was all about, she said warily, after consulting her notes, that she had noticed nothing amiss, except for some stylistic errors. Then we told her about the teacher's jibe. She said cautiously that the teacher had indeed behaved oddly at times and that she was considering the question of her professional aptitude. The principal promised to talk to the teacher, and the outcome was that the teacher apologized to Natasha in front of the class, saying that she had not meant any offense and asking her to pass the apology on to her father. Natasha's father, at the time, was already in solitary confinement at Lefortovo Prison. I can imagine how the teacher would have gloated had she known, the confirmation of her political vigilance! But nobody ever told her.

Another detail. Before my arrest, my wife ordered a dress from a seamstress, a Russian woman. When she came to collect it after the arrest, the seamstress said she would not take any money from my wife, since she must be pretty hard up as it was.

And now, in conclusion, a few words about the "curs." At the scientists' polyclinic there was a doctor (a Jew) who used to treat my children. Natasha fell ill after my arrest, and my wife rang up the clinic, asking for this doctor. She received a harsh refusal: the clinic did not service enemies of the people or members of their families. Then my wife phoned the doctor at home and asked him to come and see the sick child. He came, stayed a short time (it was a simple touch of tonsillitis), and my wife hesitantly offered him some money, fearing she might offend him. But he was not offended: he took the money without hesitation, giving no thought to my wife's hard circumstances or to the tradition according to which one physician never takes money from another (my wife is a doctor too). Unlike the seamstress, he was not overburdened with conscience. He never came again, and I am sorry I cannot remember his name.

I have cited the nationality of some of the people mentioned here just to demonstrate once again that nationality has nothing to do with ethics.

– 7 –

In Prison

LET US RETURN to the room on the ground floor of the prison where, after the doctor's examination of all the orifices of my body, I was given prison underwear to put on (another hygienic measure) and was led by a guard through some inner corridors and staircases to my cell. Passing through one of the many doors on the third floor, I was stunned at a panorama I felt I had seen before—but where? It was a square yard enclosed by four walls, four stories high. Metal netting was stretched over the yard at the level of each floor, and a gallery some two meters wide ran along the perimeter of the square on each floor. Along the edge of the gallery ran iron banisters to which the interfloor netting was attached. A multitude of doors, now closed, looked onto the gallery. They obviously led to cells. Where had I seen this before? Or was I imagining that I had seen it? After some brainracking, I recalled that I had seen it in a Soviet film about a revolt in America's Sing-Sing Prison, which ended in a mass shooting of prisoners. Probably the sets in the film had been patterned after this particular prison. Or are all prisons in the world built according to a single plan arrived at by an exchange of mutual experience?

A door was opened, and I was led into a solitary cell. Its furnishings consisted of an iron bedstead covered with a thin mattress and a little table with an aluminum bowl, an enamel mug, and a spoon—standard prisoner issue. The cell was narrow—about a meter and a half wide and no more than three meters long. In the wall opposite the door, high up near the ceiling, was a small grilled window with a sloping sill cut through the thickness of the wall. To the right of the door was a radiator, also covered by a grille, which issued barely perceptible heat. And—the cell was quite posh—opposite the bed there was a tap above a tiny semicircular sink and a cone-shaped toilet connected to the sewage system. I appreciated these modern conveniences at once: there was no traditional bucket that had to be taken out by the prisoner every day, and this small advantage made up for the smell that emanated from the toilet now and then. The walls of the cell were painted green—the symbolic color of hope, which in this case had to stand for utter hopelessness.

When the door of the cell closed behind me and I was alone, exhausted and driven to the limits of my endurance by the preceding events and two sleepless nights—it was the afternoon of the third day by then—I flopped down on the bed and was immediately introduced to the meaning of "special regime." I found out I was not alone—a watchful eye followed my every movement through the peephole in the door. The eye belonged to a woman who suddenly materialized in my cell. She wore the uniform of a prison guard, with a beret on her head and the vicious face of a dog trained to hunt people down. She growled at me: "Get up! It's forbidden to lie down in the daytime." Not yet familiar with the rules of the hotel whose guest I was, I tried to remonstrate, naively telling her that I had not slept for forty-eight hours. She was adamant. Extreme exhaustion forced me down again and again, and each time that fury burst into the cell to raise me with her bark. I decided that for this particular form of torture men were regarded as inadequate, and so women trained in the Gestapo tradition were used. Perhaps I was mistaken, but among most of the male guards (not all) there were at least some vestiges of human feeling left.

So I spent my first day in prison, tortured by fatigue, over-

whelmed by the nightmarish events, and denied the only escape physiology dictated—protective inhibition, that is, sleep.
Evening came, and a dull bulb was switched on in the ceiling. It
did not provide much light and only enhanced the nightmarish
quality of my surroundings. As I sat on my bed, I suddenly
heard rhythmical tapping on the wall. To see if I was imagining
things, I tapped back, careful not to change my sitting posture
so as not to alert the watchdog on the other side of the door. In
response came a burst of rapid tapping. But since, unlike the
well-prepared prisoners of tsarist times, I did not know the
tapping alphabet, I decided not to respond. The circumstances
of a Soviet prison, lack of any knowledge about one's neighbors,
and the possibility that the tapping was a provocation instead of
an attempt to contact a kindred soul, made one wary. My neighbor, too, soon stopped tapping.

All around me was the oppressive silence of prison, broken
only by the shuffling of the guards' feet and the clicking of the
shutter over the peephole. Some sixth sense told me that hundreds of people were immured in the stone cells of this house of
the dead. About ten o'clock in the evening (so I surmised) the
door of my cell opened and a guard entered (whom, it had
already been impressed on me, I was supposed to greet by
standing up). He was holding a scrap of paper in his hand.
"Your name?" he demanded in a whisper, for no reason that I
could see, certainly not out of consideration for other inmates. I
gave my name, also in a whisper. "Come along for interrogation!" And along I went.

But before I describe the next interrogation, I want to say a
few words about general conditions in the special-regime prison, where I landed because of my refusal to "come clean." At
6:00 a.m. they would open the little hatch in my door that
connected my cell with the outside world (food was also passed
through it), and a voice announced "Time to rise!" This meant I
was to assume a vertical position, to wash and get ready for the
next item of the regime—breakfast, which consisted of a mug
of prison "coffee," with sugar (two lumps, or two thimblefuls of

granulated sugar), and a bowl of millet gruel. The daily ration of bread (quite sufficient to keep body and soul together, by the way) was also issued in the morning. After breakfast the hours stretched out in glum meditation, interrupted by lunch—a bowl of cabbage soup, in which floated some microscopic bits of meat, and another bowl of gruel. Then the tedious hours wore on till supper—a bowl of bean or pea soup with bits of fish and a mug of weak tea. After supper came the most depressing hours, waiting for interrogation (I was called for interrogation every night with the exception of Sundays). Waiting for yet another encounter between common sense and monkey logic was unbearably depressing. At 9:30 p.m. precisely, that is, half an hour before the signal for bedtime, the guard appeared to summon me for interrogation, which went on till 5:00 in the morning. So I was left with only an hour's legitimate sleep. But I was never allowed to sleep even that much. In the first place, I returned to the cell after the interrogation in a state of feverish tension, as after a difficult duel that I could not afford to lose. I went over the questions and answers in my mind until the signal to rise in the morning was given; it often found me shaking all over. Moreover, ever solicitous of the prisoner's hygiene, the guards often made me take a shower after an interrogation, and this ate up the remaining hour. Then followed the daytime, when lying down was forbidden, and so it went, countless days without sleep. Sometimes I fell asleep during the day standing up, but my legs buckled under me and I snapped awake. If I closed my eyes when sitting down, a shout quickly followed: "Get up, open your eyes!"

There was one particularly vicious watchdog, a man with rotten teeth and a malicious glint in his eyes. Once, weak beyond measure, I dozed off while sitting on my bed and did not notice him enter the cell. He awakened me with a shout: "What's the matter, can't you see what's going on in your own cell? Want to be sent downstairs?" (a hint at the punishment cell). I tried to explain, hoping that he knew about the physiological nature of sleep from his own experience, that I had been going without sleep for many days and was therefore powerless to fight against it, that it was too strong for me. But I expect a shark would have heeded a prayer from a little fish sooner than this brute would have understood a human plea. To my explanation he gave a curt reply: "You must observe the regime. Pour cold water over your head if you're sleepy, or I'll pour it over you myself." And he tried to make the threat good then and there.

So I finally realized that this was the MGB interpretation of the word "regime." I have often been asked what regime I follow that has allowed me to preserve my intellectual capacities and relative physical strength to the age of ninety. I reply that I was on a (forced) regime only during my stay at Lefortovo. Up to that point I had believed that regime, or regimen, was a system of living, the purpose of which was to create favorable conditions for the rearing of children or for, say, the treatment of patients in hospitals, the promotion of sports skills, or the accomplishment of creative work. In the MGB version, regime was a system of suppressing will power and reason, of reducing a person to a somnambulant state when he would break down under the interrogator's questioning. Deprivation of sleep was one of the most effective elements of this regime. I cannot say how many days I went without sleep. Once I protested to my "curator." He replied: "You've been brought here to work and not to sleep." I was not so much surprised by the gist of this answer as by the use of the verb "work." I had heard it from him before too. A pretty young woman, also an MGB worker, used to drop in on my interrogator and have friendly chats with him. Once she suggested that he call it a day and go home, to which he replied, "No, I'll work with Yakov Lvovich a bit more." For him it was work, and he was paid for it, but why should I regard it as work?

In prison I developed a distaste for food. This was the kind of mentally induced loss of appetite that in some cases leads to cerebral cachexia—the wasting of the body caused by a disruption in brain function (it happens in severe mental traumas and organic lesions of the central nervous system). My prison mentors took a simpler view of it: they decided that I had gone on a hunger strike, an expression of protest that cannot be tolerated in a special-regime prison. So on the fourth or fifth day of my confinement, a stout MGB colonel bustled into my cell. He was head doctor of the prison, and he had come to persuade me to start eating. He informed me that though prison fare differed from what I was used to at home, it was still quite wholesome. He concluded his short and harsh injunction with the threat of forced feeding, paying no heed to my explanation that I was not eating only because I had no appetite. To avoid forced feeding, I stopped returning unconsumed food through the little window, but sent it down the drain. But my guards were too watchful, and one of them, who had some kindness left (I shall write more about him further on), once entered my cell as I was emptying my bowl into the toilet and said in a reproachful tone: "Why are you doing that? We see everything, you know. You must eat!" My interrogator was informed about my attitude to food, and he too reasoned with me—not for humane reasons of course—that I must eat to keep up my strength, which I was going to need. What a touching note! Thus passed my days in prison.

Sometimes sounds penetrated my cell walls. From nearby I once heard the screams of a prisoner who had obviously gone insane. They were disjointed words addressed to someone called Lyoshka. I could also hear a guard trying to reason with the madman. Several hours later, the lunatic calmed down or, what is more probable, was taken away. I still shudder at the recollection of those wild screams resounding through the silence of the prison.

From outside sometimes came the wall-shaking roar of a wind tunnel (the Zhukovsky Research Institute of Aerodynamics was close by). I heard it during my first so-called walk, several days after arrival. I had no concept then what a prison walk was. Through some passages, I was led to a quadrangle some 40 square meters in area, surrounded by tall concrete walls, with only a bit of the sky and a tower with sentry visible. As soon as I entered this pen, the wind tunnel began to roar. It was of course a coincidence but, having no experience of prison ways, I decided that I was going to be shot in that concrete box and that a siren had been switched on to muffle the shots. Not a very cheerful walk. In time I got used to the roaring and even used it for camouflage: I sat down on the bedstead and raised the collar of my coat as though to stop my ears from the noise and, with my eyes concealed from the watchdogs' vigilance, had a few minutes' doze.

Once every ten days a pushcart arrived. The vendor passed a food parcel through my door hatch: biscuits, a chunk of butter, some smoked sausage, sometimes onions, a cake of soap and cigarettes. The price was scrupulously deducted from the money confiscated during my arrest and from what my wife sent me. The balance was returned to me when I was released. I was not a smoker and once told the vendor to give my cigarettes to some other prisoner who had no money to buy them. He rejected the idea with indignation. We were not allowed to have matches, so I have no idea how the prisoners lit up.

Two other procedures that constituted part of my initiation into prisoner status were fingerprinting and photographing. For this purpose, soon after arrival, I was taken to the basement where there was a photo studio. The photographer, as in the finest studio in Moscow, helped me to assume the proper pose, asked me to button up the regulation undershirt ("It doesn't look nice opened like that"), and took my photos full face and in profile. Then he smeared my fingertips with black ink, and my prints were immortalized for the criminal archives.

But now let us return to my first summons for interrogation. The guard led me along some passages to a building that looked like an office, with wide corridors and many doors. I was taken through one of the doors into a room, where the investigator I had already met at Lubyanka was waiting for me. He wore the same haughty and contemptuous expression, but this, I later learned, was a professional mask. In actual fact, he had a lively face and was not at all haughty. He soon dropped his assumed solemnity, making up for it with another professional trait of the MGB investigator—brash familiarity born of consciousness of who holds the upper hand in the investigator-prisoner relationship.

To the right of the door stood a little table and stool, both fastened to the floor. To the left, at a distance, was a big desk at which my investigator was ensconced. He was obviously proud of the appurtenances of his office because once, in the presence of several of his young colleagues, he asked my opinion of it: "What office do you like better, this one or the one where the colonel interrogated you yesterday?" (I shall speak later about that interrogation.) I answered that most of all I liked my unpretentious office in the pathology department of the First Gradskaya Hospital. This caused them to exchange puzzled looks. Apparently they were already aware of the new turn the case was taking, and my answer had startled them.

The investigator told me to sit down on the stool and proceeded to inform me that my case was in his sole charge and that any questions or requests I might have must be addressed to him, for their solution depended upon him. The implication of these words seemed to be that I belonged to him like some inanimate object and that therefore, if I knew what was good for me, I would behave. At this point I want to say a few words about my investigator. He introduced himself as deputy head of the investigation department. I have no idea why I was so honored. Other investigators often came to ask his advice, and I watched them with curiosity. They were all young people, recent graduates of law schools (I even knew some of their professors). They looked like ordinary enough people with normal human faces; there was nothing brutal in their appearances. I was surprised at this dissonance between their looks and the vile work they were doing. But often the outward brutality of such officers is mere theatrics; many of the most sadistic and ferocious Gestapo men had angelic faces. One particular investigator who often dropped in, a young man suffering from furunculosis, was in charge of the case of Miron Vovsi's wife. I asked him to give her my regards (which he did) and pleaded that he should not torment her too cruelly. He denied the fact of tormenting, then asked me why I was staring at him. I said that he reminded me of one of my students and that his looks were at variance with his duties. "Why, are we a different brand of people?" he asked. They really did regard themselves as people like all others and, I imagine, might have been quite decent in another world and time. My investigator had several facets to his personality. He was shrewd and easy-going, with a smattering of knowledge in literature and biology. Strange as it may seem, I harbor no hatred for him. And I feel grateful for his occasional manifestations of humanity and for those chats on outside subjects he sometimes permitted, which were like a breath of fresh air in my solitary confinement. Sometimes I imagined he felt sympathy for me in my plight. But for all that, he was an MGB investigator and did his job conscientiously, that is, he tried to make me admit something that had never been and to give a tendentious interpretation to that which had been.

After he informed me of the rules of our relationship, I asked him where I was. "In Lefortovo Prison." I was gripped by fear. Lefortovo had a terrible reputation, the worst of all the Moscow prisons. It was believed that nobody ever left it alive, that the very fact of confinement there was tantamount to a death sentence. My wife had a dread horror of the place. Fortunately, she did not know I was in Lefortovo; she believed I was being held in Lubyanka. Later she told me that, had she known where I was, she would not have been able to endure it.

It is difficult for me to compare the prisons since I spent only twenty-four hours at Lubyanka (more on this later). The only difference I noticed was that at Lubyanka a waitress in a white apron and headdress brought my food into the cell, and that the cell did not have the modern conveniences of Lefortovo, which I prized very highly. But Lina Stern, who spent almost three years at Lubyanka and was then brought, for purposes of intimidation, to Lefortovo, where she stayed for twenty days, described the latter as hell. So one needs a starting point for comparison. I had none, and I was glad to be spending my confinement in a solitary cell. I preferred being alone to being among people I did not know, some of them possibly informers. One of the most feared features of Lefortovo's regime—solitary confinement—was something I had no objection to in the circumstances. Of course I have no idea how I would have felt if my confinement had gone on for years.

Thus the wakeful nightly sessions began, with a respite on Sundays when my investigator, like all Soviet citizens, enjoyed his constitutional right to rest. After elucidating the terms of our relationship, the investigator supplied another important piece of information. Before starting the interrogation, he told me in a cheery tone that I was in no danger of being shot. I saw this as a peculiar start. In normal legal practice, the investigator's role is to establish guilt, while the punishment is decided by the court. In Soviet jurisprudence during the Stalin era, things were stood on their head, and the sentence was known from the beginning. It might have been, however, that my curator gave me this assurance in hopes of loosening my tongue. It was necessary because the articles of the Soviet Criminal Code I was arrested under (58.8, 58.10, and 58.11) all stipulated capital punishment. I was supposed to have committed my crimes not on my own but as a member of an organization (article 58.11). The assurance was supposed to encourage me to divulge my own participation and to denounce others. Soon, though, my investigator decided to revoke the assurance. Not that his promise actually reassured me: I saw no reason why an exception should be made in my case. I knew where I was and in whose hands, and the meaning of those articles of the Criminal Code had been explained to me. Article 58.10—anti-Soviet propaganda; article 58.8—active terrorist activities; article 58.11—membership in a terrorist organization, which heightened the severity of the first two crimes. Generally, article 58 of the Criminal Code was the worst, and it accounted for most death sentences during the years of Stalinist terror.

When my investigator realized that he had failed to obtain not only an admission of my participation in organized terrorist acts but even an admission that there had been such acts, he declared: "You have the reputation of being a clever person, but you behave like a fool." Recently I heard something like this from my eight-year-old granddaughter, after I had paid a drunkard of a carpenter for work in advance. He drank up the money and never appeared to finish the job. The child repeated the investigator's description almost word for word: "Grandad seems so intelligent, but he acts like a fool." (This time I deserved it, so I was not offended.) The investigator held Miron Vovsi up to me as an example: "Vovsi behaves like a clever man, and will perhaps escape with his life, but your behavior is stupid." At this I reminded him of his own assurance that I was in no danger of the firing squad. "That depends on the people's will," he said. I had no doubt that "the people" would want executions. This was confirmed, incidentally, by my investigator and his colleagues, who discussed the ritual of the forthcoming executions in my presence. Since the promise to spare my life bore no fruit, he decided to achieve his end by threatening execution. I must confess, however, that I was unable to see this threat in real terms. For me it was an abstraction that would have become real, I expect, only at the actual moment of execution. This psychological negation of death may not be a personal characteristic so much as a manifestation of life's vital force in general.

To proceed with the nocturnal sessions: it is impossible to convey their phantasmagoric character in the coherent shape of a narration. Over many, many nights, one and the same subject was rehashed again and again, with numerous digressions and startling out-of-the blue questions apparently prepared by my investigator beforehand. I expect their purpose was to confuse the man being questioned and to catch him in a lie. The same aim was apparently pursued through the endless repetition of questions in the same area, so that a chink might appear in my denials that could be used against me. Such interrogational tricks are commonly known from detective novels, where the questioner pits his brain against the man he questions. I would not undertake to give a comparative assessment of my intellect and my investigator's, but the MGB men had formed a high opinion of my mental powers. The character given me by informers, with which my investigator acquainted me, said that I was an outstanding scientist whose name was well known in the USSR and abroad, that I was clever and cunning, and that in questioning me an investigator must have all his wits about him. To this I replied that his informers had fatally overestimated my role both in the criminal and the scientific world.

The questions discussed during the nocturnal sessions, despite all the confusion, fell into two main categories: (1) Jewish bourgeois nationalism and (2) participation in terrorist acts perpetrated by the organization of killer doctors. Just as during our first meeting at Lubyanka, the investigator began by suggesting that I tell him about my crimes. This I could not do, since I did not even understand what was meant by Jewish bourgeois nationalism. The investigator helped out on this, reading aloud the part about me in the deposition of one of the prominent medical men they had arrested. I was described as a protector of the Jewish employees at the Institute of Morphology, who were persecuted in one way or another. This was quite true, for I had indeed tried to protect those whose nationality was their only flaw. Now my eyes were opened, and I understood why I was classed as a Jewish bourgeois nationalist and an enemy of the Soviet people. It appeared that finding endless fault with Jewish research fellows and placing them under fear and stress, as was openly done by Professor Zilov, the head of personnel at the Academy of Medical Sciences, was not a crime, despite the article in the Criminal Code that carried punishment for antisemitism and was occasionally enforced in the 1920s. The real crime now was to protect those who were insulted and persecuted because of their nationality, and even to sympathize with them was a crime, called Jewish bourgeois nationalism. I did not deny the charge, nor did I bother to conceal my views on the subject, since I did not consider them criminal. Generally, throughout the investigation, I followed a clear-cut line: to admit to views and actions that were in no way reprehensible (in my opinion) and to deny everything that had never happened.

This line seemed incomprehensible to the investigator: why should I admit to and even expound some of my views, which were punishable according to article 58, and deny other views and actions to which the same article applied? He simply could not understand that I never lied, although I did not go so far as to air all my opinions on Soviet reality. And these opinions, especially in the preceding few years, were despondent indeed. But having launched on the path of Jewish bourgeois nationalism, I went on at length and in detail about the numerous cases of discrimination against Jews in various fields of life—cases of which I had first-hand knowledge.

The next session began with the following announcement from my investigator: "You say Jews have been refused admission to some higher educational establishments. This is quite possible, but not because they were Jews but because they did not conform to the strict social requirements for enrollment in that particular institute." I suppose he was told to say this by superiors who reviewed all the previous interrogations of those accused. After hearing this explanation, I told him that I found it very interesting and that at my trial—if ever there was one— I would quote him as having said that selection by social origins at our higher educational establishments had now been replaced by selection according to nationality. Apparently stung by my remark, he exclaimed heatedly, "You are misrepresenting my words!" I smiled at this—it was somewhat amusing, considering my situation.

Then I told him that, as deputy director of the Institute of Morphology, I was informed by the personnel director of the institute that she had been instructed to keep Jews from obtaining employment at the institute. I also cited, as an example of state-promoted antisemitism and not by local initiative (which had been even less completely eradicated), the episode of the publication of a reference book on the histological diagnosis of tumors. This was a much-needed book, considering the vital importance of correct characterization of tumors, especially in biopsies. There was no such work in our medical literature and, at my initiative, a Russian translation of *Identification of Tumors* by the major American authority on the morphology of tumors, Nathan Chandler Foot, was published in Moscow in 1950, with my foreword and under my editorship. It sold out immediately and soon became a bibliographical rarity, which pathologists cherished and kept under lock and key. Most pathologists were grateful to me for organizing the publication of the book, but there were quite a few who expressed (out of my hearing) displeasure at this "cosmopolitan" action. They even spread rumors that I had been called on the carpet for my work on Foot's book.

Still it became increasingly obvious that a similar reference book written by Soviet authors was needed. The Leningrad Institute of Oncology and the head of its pathology department, Mikhail Glazunov, an authority on tumors, were charged with compiling the work. The field of tumor morphology is vast. One author, however knowledgeable, cannot cover the infinite number of tumors, the structure of which varies according to the organ where the tumor develops, its maturity, its benignity or malignity, and so on. Thus pathologists specialize in a particular branch of oncology. Glazunov himself, although a broad specialist, was mainly known as an expert on female genitalia. He decided to put together a team of authors with experience in various kinds of tumors, among them the Academician Lev Shabad, a prominent theoretician of oncology, and myself. We both agreed to contribute to the book, listed sections we would write and provide illustrations for, and received letters from Glazunov with thanks for our cooperation and confirmation of the sections we named and their length. This happened in 1951. We never heard from Glazunov again.

Then on January 6, 1953—I remember the date precisely—I met Glazunov at a meeting of the Society of Pathologists. We greeted each other and exchanged a few polite words, but he never mentioned the reference book. It was as if there had never been any mention of my making a contribution to it. I sat beside him at the session and asked him the purpose of his visit to Moscow. He said he had come to conclude a contract with Medgiz Publishers on the tumor reference book, and again said not a word about my own part in it. I saw how matters stood but decided to force a confirmation from him. So I asked him: "Shall I get down to work then?" Glazunov made a vague gesture, the meaning of which, however, was perfectly clear. When I asked "What about Shabad?" he said curtly: "No exceptions allowed." After the session he told me exactly what had happened. When he came to the director of Medgiz, Vasily Banshchikov (chief editor of the publishing house, Academician Anatoly Strukov, was also present at the conversation), Banshchikov crossed out Shabad's and my name from the list of authors (we were the only two Jews on the list). When Glazunov objected that this jeopardized the quality and possible publication of the book, Banshchikov simply ignored his words. Glazunov then went to see the president of the Academy of Medical Sciences, Nikolai Anichkov, who, as Glazunov put it, "was no happier about it than I was." The book was not published, and for the next twenty-five years Soviet pathologists had only scarce, dog-eared copies of Foot's book to use.

I told my investigator this story, which demonstrated the discrimination against Jewish scientists unconcealed, in this case, by any fig leaves. The investigator was incensed. But his anger was aimed not at Medgiz Publishers, who had committed the brazenly antisemitic action, but at Glazunov, who had dared to tell me about it. He threatened to take action against him, but I didn't think that Glazunov was in any real danger. No one had demanded a pledge of secrecy from him, and he was not obliged to keep quiet about the incident, especially since its deeper wellsprings were clear to all and sundry. President Anichkov had asked the Central Committee if the literary ostracism of the two Jewish authors concerned only their contribution to the manual on tumors. He received a categorical reply: it meant complete banishment from publishing.

While I am on the subject, let me relate one incident that also did not appear in the materials of the investigation but provides yet another graphic illustration of the atmosphere in the medical world as the Doctors' Plot was being hatched. Back during World War II, my textbook *A Course in Pathology* was published. It was reprinted several times in Moscow and in the Ukraine, Georgia, and Estonia, also in Bulgaria and China. Another edition of the textbook came out in 1950. In May 1953, soon after my release, Medgiz Publishers sent me, simply for information, a manuscript review of the last edition written by A. Yukhlov and A. Eingorn, both with candidate degrees in medicine. I had never met the former and knew nothing about him, but I knew Eingorn. When I was deputy director of the Institute of Morphology, he had been a graduate student, working in Strukov's laboratory. He had the reputation of being a man of less than average ability and very little dedication. After defending his thesis, he was mobilized into the army to teach in a military medical school.

The review written by these two luminaries was dated December 1952. A special need for it had obviously arisen, two years after the latest edition had come out. As Eingorn later confirmed, they had been ordered to write it. The authors really exerted themselves, even as to the size of the review (eleven typewritten pages). As to content, it was a denunciation rather than a review. The authors did not feel constrained to examine the actual text of the book. Their device was time-honored: they ascribed to the author things he never said and then went on to rip him to shreds. But still their ignorance was flagrant, both in their analysis of the book and in their recommendations to the author. Theoretically they proceeded from the pseudo-scientific conceptions enforced at the time. But those who ordered the review did not care about science; they only wanted to demonstrate with a semblance of objectivity that the author of the book was a follower of Virchow, then in disrepute in official Soviet science, and that he preached harmful ideas and methods in his book. I kept this review as a document of the epoch. (My book ran through several more editions after 1953.)

In 1954, a national conference of pathologists was held in Leningrad. During a recess, two people in uniform approached me in the foyer (one was a lieutenant-colonel and the other a major). In one of them I recognized Eingorn. He greeted me with an expression of pure joy on his face and introduced his companion—Dr. Yukhlov. I said I knew the name and the man's face lit up—he imagined that I remembered it from scientific literature. I was quick to disappoint him, saying that the only place I had seen his name was on the review of my textbook. Both looked embarrassed. I told them, quite amiably, that I was grateful to them for their advice that I should shake off the influence of Virchowianism, while I for my part advised them to acquaint themselves with Virchow's works if they wanted to get anywhere in pathology. With this, our "reunion" ended.

Five years later I learned the story of the writing of the review. At that time, on the invitation of Academician Alexander Bakulev, I accepted the post of head of the pathomorphology laboratory at the Institute of Cardiac Surgery he had set up. (It is now named after him.) I needed specialists for my laboratory and placed an ad in a newspaper about a competition for the jobs of senior and junior research fellows. Suddenly whom did I see but Eingorn entering my office and informing me that he had been sent by Strukov. Eingorn told me that he had asked for a discharge from the army, would soon return to Moscow, and would like to get a job as a senior research fellow in my laboratory. I was not particularly surprised by his shamelessness, but *he* was—by my flat refusal. I told him that far from supporting his request I would, if he decided to take part in the competition, do everything in my power not to have him employed in my laboratory. To his puzzled question why (he obviously expected me to receive him with open arms), I gave him my reasons. They were, first and foremost, his poor qualifications, which had been low enough in his graduate years and which had certainly become lower still during his many years in the army. Then I said that I had not forgotten his despicable review of my book, knowing full well that at the time such a review meant the author's scientific, if not physical, liquidation. Eingorn told me how the review was written, fully convinced that he was not in the least to blame, since he simply executed an order given him by Strukov, chief editor at Medgiz. In the fall of 1952, Strukov had summoned him and ordered him and his head of department, Yukhlov, to write a negative review of my textbook. He told Eingorn what the main points of the review should be. When the review was ready, the two of them were again summoned to Moscow, and the director of Medgiz, Banshchikov, said it would be published immediately in *Arkhiv patologii*. The galleys of the journal arrived from the printer after I had already been arrested. By the rules of the time, the name of a person who had been arrested could not be mentioned in any context, not even a negative one. He was to be consigned to oblivion; his works were removed from the libraries; no references to them were allowed in academic papers and their possession was regarded as reprehensible, tantamount to possession of illegal literature. After my arrest, the review was canceled from the issue. So only my arrest protected me from having this abomination published. Despite this explanation, I granted Eingorn no amnesty. And I don't think he ever understood what he had done wrong: after all, he had not written the review of his own free will.

My scientific convictions often came up for discussion during the prison interrogations. The investigator was well informed. My two-volume dossier contained not only informers' reports but also summaries of my speeches. Once, for instance, the investigator exclaimed with righteous anger: "Do you realize how low you have sunk? To compare Boshian, the greatest scientist of our time, to a dead horse!" I was reminded of a forgotten incident, which had actually taken place at a conference of medical scientists at the university. A major functionary of the Ministry of Health declared, holding Boshian's thin booklet in his hand: "Old microbiology is dead. Here is new microbiology for you." I had read the booklet: the charlatan Boshian, on the basis of crude experiments, had trampled Pasteur's work into the mud. Subsequently he was exposed for the ignoramus he was; his high rank and awards were taken from him and he disappeared from view. Well, discussing Boshian's discovery, I said: "I will not touch on the virological aspect of this book, for I am no authority on virology. But the author here cites autopsies of dead horses, and, as a pathologist, I must say that these autopsy reports were not written by any kind of pathologist, but in all probability by the horse itself, on the brink of death. These are the ravings of a dying horse." That, to quote my investigator, was how low I had sunk.

Since among the incriminating evidence taken from my apartment was a photograph of Olga Lepeshinskaya, the investigator asked me: "Why do you keep a photograph of Lepeshinskaya if you have nothing but contempt for her theory?" I replied that the photograph had been a present to me from Lepeshinskaya herself, of which he could assure himself by reading her friendly inscription on the back. I had been friends with Lepeshinskaya for many years, had great respect for her as a veteran Bolshevik and a biologist, and I myself took that photograph at my dacha. A complete break occurred between us after a heated argument—again at my dacha—in the course of which I told her in no uncertain terms what I thought of her ridiculous theory of the "vital substance." To her credit, Lepeshinskaya never tried to retaliate in any way. The story of my relations with Lepeshinskaya and my attitude toward her theory received an unexpected sequel in the city of Frunze (Kirghizia), some six thousand kilometers from Moscow, and the investigator obviously knew about the sequel and used it to complement the picture of my "scientific heresy."

A good friend of mine, Veniamin Kaplan, a specialist on the history of the United States, told me about the Frunze incident. In 1948 he published a book on the postwar history of the United States. Some "cultural leader" took exception, and a devastating review of the book appeared in a party periodical. As a result, Kaplan was packed off to Frunze to teach political economy at the local medical college (not too harsh a punishment by the standards of those times). Since he was teaching in a medical college, he got a good introduction to the mores of the medical world. As is often the case, people in the provinces tried to keep abreast of every new trend in medicine that was initiated "at the top" and tended to be, as the saying goes, more catholic than the pope. One such relevant novelty (besides the ever relevant "Stalin is the great coryphaeus of medical science") was Lepeshinskaya's epoch-making discovery. Professors were obliged to discuss it at every lecture, and the college administration and party organization sent special observers to the lectures to see that the professors toed the line. Kaplan was also forced to act as such an observer. He made friends with many professors at the medical college, among them the professor of histology, B. The latter, like all the rest, began every lecture with adulations of Lepeshinskaya and her discoveries. His specialty, as a matter of fact, made this more required of him than the others. But in private talks he told Kaplan his real opinion of these discoveries as so much nonsense, the product of crass ignorance. Kaplan reproached him for scientific hypocrisy and duplicity and cited as an example of scientific integrity my public utterings on the subject. He also repeated my application of a rather ribald Russian saying to the commotion over Lepeshinskaya's discovery: "Not only have they made candy of this shit, but they keep pushing it into our mouths and demanding that we express our delight at the taste."

Kaplan was arrested in Frunze, about the same time I was

arrested in Moscow. Before this, many professors at the medical college were summoned to the local branch of the MGB and informed that there was irrefutable proof that he was spying for American intelligence and would soon be arrested. They were also asked—to ensure that all aspects of his anti-Soviet activities were exposed—if they could supply any additional compromising materials. Some refused, saying that they knew nothing disparaging about Kaplan. One professor paid with his life for this refusal, dying of a heart attack during a party meeting at which his unprincipled stand was discussed. Professor B., however, cooperated. He informed the MGB that Kaplan regularly listened to the Voice of America and had spoken insultingly of Lepeshinskaya's discoveries. And at this point, he cited my assessment of Lepeshinskaya's work, quoting it verbatim and naming the source. This was regarded as an insult not only to the "great scientist" but also to the high-placed bodies that decreed her glorification. So my ribald evaluation was documented by B.'s deposition.

Kaplan was brought to trial after Stalin's death. He was sentenced to a term of eight years in prison. The subsequent fate of my evaluation is interesting. A year later, Kaplan was brought back to Frunze for a retrial. The local party leadership, in the person of Razzakov, secretary of the Central Committee of the Communist Party of Kirghizia, put a great deal of pressure on the investigators entrusted with reconsidering the case—for it was Razzakov who approved (and perhaps even ordered) the arrest of the old professor. Kaplan's rehabilitation would have dealt a blow to the authority of this satrap. In view of these circumstances, a special investigator was sent from Moscow. (Razzakov was soon removed from his post.) The Moscow investigator began to summon, one after another, all those who gave testimony against Kaplan. Almost all took it back, pleading that they had given it under duress. B. also took back some of his testimony, but insisted on the authenticity of two pieces of it: the listening to the Voice of America and the "shit candy." The Moscow investigator apparently had a clear enough idea by then of the composition of Lepeshinskaya's scientific candy, though the news had not yet reached Frunze. Obviously he also knew that Rapoport had been released and fully rehabilitated. At any rate, the investigator told B. in the presence of Kaplan: "Professor Rapoport acts according to his convictions, and you say one thing publicly and something very different behind people's backs." So B. was put to shame and the candy rehabilitated. The case of Kaplan was reconsidered, he was rehabilitated, and his party membership restored. He went on to write three more fine historical monographs.

This entire episode might appear ridiculous if it did not have such grim connotations. It shows what the Ministry of State Security wasted money and human energy on, instead of protecting the security of the state.

At interrogation sessions, I discovered that I had a rich criminal biography from a scientific point of view. The investigators knew not only about my attitude to the discoveries of Lepeshinskaya and Boshian, but also about what I had said about Virchowianism, my opposition to the prophets of "a new trend in pathology," my struggle against "neurological despotism" in medicine, and my support for Lina Stern. The investigators also regarded me as an active opponent of Pavlov's teaching, but in fact I only opposed the vulgarization of his teaching by paltry imitators. After enumerating all my scientific and methodological sins, the investigator reassured me that they did not fall into the category of actions penalized by the Criminal Code. Apparently he thought that I had enough real crimes on my conscience, so there was no need to add these to confuse matters. If the need arose, however, these heresies could have been transformed into dire political crimes, as had been done in the case of geneticists, microbiologists, writers, poets, actors, artists, and so on. In my case, the scientific sins were given the role of general background. As my investigator declared, they were only important inasmuch as they helped to reveal my general anti-Soviet stance—that of a vehement enemy of advanced Soviet science and a defender of Virchow's and Stern's reactionary teachings. This was the MGB interpretation of my quixotic struggle against ignoramuses and mercenaries in science.

But let us return to the interrogation sessions. Each began with the following dialogue:

"Well?"

"Well what?"

"Talk!"

"What about?"

"You know yourself."

"I have nothing to tell you—nothing that you want."

This distasteful exchange was a prelude to every session; the very thought that I was going to be run through the same gauntlet made me feel as though somebody had twisted my gut around his finger and was winding it tighter and tighter. After several fruitless "Wells," the investigator would glance into my fat dossier and toss me a lead. So we would begin to discuss Jewish bourgeois nationalism. Among the evidence against me on this score were reports by informers, testimony of the other persons involved in the case, and my own statements about my reaction to what I in my blindness regarded as state-sponsored antisemitism.

I cannot recall how many nights were spent in chewing the cud of Jewish bourgeois nationalism. Each session had the same finale in the shape of a record, or protocol, in standard literary form, which I was supposed to sign. In the very first such protocol, I noticed in its introductory "passport section," the words "formerly a CPSU member." I objected to the adverb, saying that nobody had expelled me from the party. The investigator explained to me that I had been expelled in my absence.

This was a clear infringement of the party rules, according to which no decision concerning a member can be taken without his participation or, the more so, in his absence. It appears I was expelled from the party by the Central Committee while still enjoying my freedom, however ephemeral. The party organization of the Tarasevich Institute, upon hearing of my arrest and not knowing that I had already been expelled, hastened to add its own bit and expelled me from the party once more. But how could I, a prisoner, protest against this double violation of the rules?

In the interrogation record, my explanations and "admissions" were embellished to make them sound like real criminal acts. For example, my assertion about discrimination practiced against Jews in the matter of employment and "redundance" dismissals was recorded like this: "Full of wild fury and brutal hatred for the Soviet system, I slandered Soviet reality, asserting that Jews are discriminated against in employment and dismissals" (this may not be a verbatim rendering, but I vouch for the general style). In other words, the investigator dramatized the least fact to give it the appearance of a horrible act. Just think of it: wild fury, brutal hatred, slander—how could such a monster be allowed to tread Soviet soil? Off with his head!

Here is another example of the investigator's translation of a fact of my life. After demobilization in the spring of 1945, I did not return to the Second Medical Institute, where I had been professor of pathology and deputy director for scientific research and matriculation, but took a job at the Institute of Morphology of the Academy of Medical Sciences. At the same time, I resumed my duties at the First Gradskaya Hospital (under Topchan), which also housed my laboratory for the Institute of Morphology. This fact was given the following rendering in the protocol, which I refused to sign, demanding correction: "After demobilization I *decided* not to return to the Second Medical Institute, but *arranged* with the Jewish bourgeois nationalist Topchan *to continue* my activities at the First Gradskaya Hospital." I protested the distortions aimed at creating an impression of collusion in transferring my criminal activities to the Gradskaya and at discrediting Topchan. To this my investigator, with the most innocent of expressions, protested that the record simply repeated the facts: "Surely in order to return to the First Gradskaya Hospital you had to make arrangements, Topchan *is* a Jewish bourgeois nationalist, and any kind of job can also be considered activities of a sort," he remonstrated.

Occasionally my investigator interspersed "comic interludes" in the course of the interrogation. He asked me: "What is Kogan's name and patronymic?"

"Boris Borisovich," I replied. There was a burst of mirth:

"Ha-ha-ha! Boris Borisovich indeed! You mean Borukh-Berko-Haimovich!"

"Throughout our acquaintance I knew and addressed him as Boris Borisovich, and I never had occasion to look at his passport."

"Incidentally," the investigator continued, "according to your passport, your name is Yakov Lvovich, and all Moscow knows you as such. Yet from one of your documents [he meant my birth certificate, issued in 1898 by a rabbi in Simferopol] it is obvious that your father's name was not Lev."

"That's right," I said calmly, "my father's full name is quite complicated: Shamai-Leibovich Ioselevich Shabsovich, but in everyday life everybody called him Lev Iosifovich. If you want to address me as Yakov Shamai-Leibovich Ioselevich Shabsovich—you are welcome, twist your tongue as much as you like, I have no objection."

There was no reply. Then followed one of those questions that came out of the blue!

"Why did you refuse to rent a room to Barg?"

Hereby, as they say, hangs a tale. In the fall of 1952 after our elder daughter Naomi went to work in Toropets, there remained only the three of us (my wife, my schoolgirl daughter, and myself) in a big four-room flat. Money was rather short at the time, and we decided to take a lodger. Our friends recommended an acquaintance of theirs, an historian named Barg, who had moved to Moscow from Lvov, which had been part of Poland until 1939. However, the need to be constantly on our guard lest the MGB gave a warped interpretation to a contact with somebody from abroad finally made us decide against letting a room to a former Polish citizen. We informed our friends about our decision over the telephone. Still this fact, like many others, did receive a warped interpretation at the MGB. I explained the reason for our refusal, and when the investigator expressed doubt, I said that they had themselves instilled in Soviet citizens the fear of contacts with foreigners. But he chose to ascribe our refusal to some different, more sinister, cause.

Another out-of-the-blue question was: "Why didn't you name Etinger among your friends?" I did not at once realize he was referring to the list made out by the MGB during their attempt to recruit me nearly two years before. I said I had probably forgotten, and again the investigator did not believe me and insisted that the omission was intentional. This time he was quite right. Yakov Etinger was a talkative man who loved to discuss politics—with anybody and in any company. And he was far from careful in airing his views. The MGB certainly knew about this, since he did not hesitate to utter heresies even during his rounds of the wards in the presence of retinue and patients alike. The MGB did not require my information about his utterances, but I did not want them to pester me on this score. This episode shows, incidentally, that in the MGB's secret dossiers, every little fact was used against the person concerned. My particular dossier, I learned during the investigation and after my release, had been compiled over a period of many years. Once my investigator read me a long list of Jewish medical professors, beginning with the names Pevzner and Zbarsky, and asked me which of them I knew personally. I knew almost everybody, since the Moscow medical world is not big, and those were prominent names. What the purpose of that list was will forever remain a secret of the MGB, but the very fact of its existence is significant. Did they mean to destroy all of those people?

I was also taught several lessons about the principles of Soviet jurisprudence, which were laid down by that expert, Andrey Vyshinsky. I asked my investigator why they needed my admission of the crimes they imputed to me if I was considered guilty of them even before my arrest, and since sentence had already been passed. The investigator explained to me quite willingly that an admission on the part of the accused constituted "presumption of guilt." I knew that "presumption of guilt" is regarded as the most pernicious fallacy in the criminal codes of all nations. Then I inquired what was meant by "anti-Soviet assemblages" in which I allegedly had taken part. The investigator explained that this was also Vyshinsky's definition. "An assemblage" was a group of people, which might consist of as few as two persons, who had no definite plan for anti-Soviet activities but who discussed matters of a counterrevolutionary nature. "An organization" (a higher step in anti-Sovietism) already had a program and plan of counterrevolutionary activities.

After spending many days on proving my Jewish bourgeois nationalism, my investigator exclaimed in extreme annoyance: "What kind of materials are these? Haim was dismissed from his job, Abram was refused employment—I could have found out all this at any trade-union committee. I need a different kind of evidence." I said that I could only give materials that could indeed be obtained from any trade-union committee: I had no others to offer. Nevertheless, this inadequate evidence was regarded as sufficient to pronounce me guilty according to the death-dealing articles of the code.

Now the investigation entered the next stage—my participation in the terrorist activities of doctors. Actually, there was no distinct demarcation line between the two stages in the course of the investigation, but my attitude to the two charges was different. While I made no attempt to deny the real thoughts and actions that by MGB logic made me a Jewish bourgeois nationalist, I flatly denied terrorism, and not only my own participation in it but the very possibility of such actions on the part of the other doctors who had been arrested. I asserted that I knew them all to be first-rate doctors, dedicated to medicine and incapable of doing intentional harm to their patients. The investigator, apparently tired of my stubbornness, decided to break it with the following question: "While still at large, did you read the Tass statement of January 13, 1953?" This statement alleged that all the accused had admitted their guilt. I said

I did not believe it. There was a stream of violent abuse interrupted by: "Do you imply that this is a provocation of the MGB?"

Retribution came the next day. In a departure from the usual procedure, I was summoned for interrogation in the daytime, before lunch. I saw my investigator in the now familiar office at a strange hour. Instead of the usual "Well?" there was a harsh question: "Are you going to talk or not?" I gave my customary negative answer. There was a sharp command: "Get up! Put your hands behind your back!" I heard a metallic click, and my hands were tightly manacled: a guard who had entered the room noiselessly had handcuffed me.

It is hard to describe the design of these handcuffs, for they were quite different from the handcuffs we see in films, which look like two smooth bracelets joined with a chain. In comparison with mine, those are innocent toys. I do not know whether the design of the handcuffs used in Soviet special-regime prisons was ever patented, but I imagine that I will not be divulging a state secret if I describe them. The central part of the handcuffs consists of a flat square lock with a side of about 8 centimeters and some 2 centimeters thick. To the lock are joined two parts of movable crescent-shaped claws. The overlapping edges of the claws are serrated in such a way that, when the two claws are snapped together, the notches on one enter the grooves on the other and the wrists are locked in a complete bracelet and joined by the lock. Now an important detail: if you instinctively jerk your hands, the notches on the claws shift into the next groove—but only in one direction—and make the bracelets tighter. Can you imagine the effect? An awkward movement, a click, and the grip on the wrists is tightened. After a while your hands become horribly swollen.

The handcuffs were removed only three times a day for five to ten minutes—for meals and the performance of the natural bodily functions. For the night the manacles were moved to the front and locked on the stomach. These operations with the handcuffs were carried out by the guards. The degree of sadism they exhibited in the process differentiated them into curs and human beings. There was one particular cur who made a point of twisting my arms every time he pulled my hands behind my back; this was particularly painful to my left arm, which had been fractured during the war and had only a limited range of movement when drawn back. The cur made the handcuffs so tight that they would bite into my flesh. The more human guard put the handcuffs on with a guilty expression and he once even said to me, although he certainly had no right to (generally, the guards were not supposed to enter into conversations with prisoners): "They make us do it, you know!" He said it in reply to my request to make the bracelets looser, and he went on to explain that if they were too loose they would chafe my wrists until I developed sores. He did his best to choose the optimal diameter.

After being awarded the handcuffs, I was posted back to my cell. I was stunned. The handcuffs were a rude intervention into my dreary, oppressive but by then familiar routine—a new and undoubtedly sinister feature. I had been manacled not because I might attempt to escape: it was not only additional torment but also a symbol of the low status of a prisoner, involving "additional restrictions." I felt debased, violated, and helpless and, in a frenzy of despair, began to beat my head against the wall of the cell. The guards burst in and restrained me, saying: "Do you want to knock down the wall? Want a spell downstairs?" (the punishment cell).

The interrogations resumed, and now there was more browbeating than before. At the next nocturnal session, still shaken and worked up, I demanded that the handcuffs be removed. The investigator refused, intimating that the measure had not been his doing. He even said: "Do you think I like seeing you in handcuffs? It's your own fault."

One dreary night after another, he went on trying to drag out an admission of crimes I had never committed. I remained steadfast in my denials, despite the Tass statement of January 13, despite the handcuffs and the expectation of worse things to come. According to the legend fabricated by the MGB, the killer doctors had great respect for me and shared with me the secrets of their methods of doing away with illustrious patients, while my task was to conceal their crimes when I performed autopsies. Others killed, and I covered up their crimes—such was the role assigned to me by the MGB in the Doctors' Plot.

The investigator constructed a pattern of thinking that was supposed to have led me and the other killer doctors to conclude that there was a need for terrorist actions. This is how he reasoned on our behalf: "Jews are being persecuted, denied jobs, exposed to hardships. Something must be done, we have to fight against it all!" And the only possible method of struggle could be terror, the killing of those who had initiated and directed the persecution of the Jews. This is what he wanted me to admit. I pointed out to him that the organization of killer doctors was supposed to include some Russians too—Vinogradov, Vasilenko, Zelenin, Yegorov, and others. What moved them, I asked, what could they have been fighting, these prosperous and respected people who were not subject to any racial discrimination? He ignored this argument altogether. As I have mentioned, the man in the street believed that they were secretly Jews. And, indeed, why else should they be sharing the fate of the Jewish professors? Anyway, what is a Soviet Jew? How is he to be distinguished from other nationalities if he does not know Yiddish (many have never even heard it spoken), if he regards Russian as his mother tongue, has been brought up on Russian literature and culture? It appears that in defining the concept of "Jew" we must proceed from the rule of opposites: a Jew is somebody who is subject to antisemitism. In the light of this definition, it was quite logical to regard the Russian doctors purported to be participants in the plot as Jews, since they were victims of antisemitism. There is nothing paradoxical about this interpretation: antisemitism, after all, is an inherently animalistic feeling, akin to cannibalism, projected onto Jews. Over the centuries, antisemites have tried to build a doctrine on the basis of this feeling. As we know, the most consistent and thorough in their genocidal interpretation were the Nazis.

A few words apropos Nazism. My erudite investigator once

asked me if I knew that Nazi doctrine had been created by Jews as well. Even Goebbels would have never ascribed Nazi doctrine to "refined Jewish intellectualism" (the contemptuous formula he used to describe many achievements of world culture that the Nazis regarded as alien to them). I said in reply: "It is quite possible." My curator stared at me in amazement—he must have expected a burst of indignant denials—and asked why I thought so. I said: "Many major social doctrines such as Christianity and Marxism were developed by Jews. So why not Nazism?" He did not pursue the subject, but this twist of reasoning on the part of the MGB to justify antisemitism speaks for itself.

The investigator's twisted logic fell flat. However much he reiterated the cue, "But you had to fight," I refused to admit any participation in terrorist activities. Even then I was not sure what disgusted me more—the handcuffs or listening to those imbecilities. Also I had to be on my guard all the time to parry concrete accusations with common sense, although there was as much point in my attempts to reason with him as in trying to explain to a deaf-mute the difference between a frog's croaking and a nightingale's song. I got so worked up during these sessions, it cost me so much strain to watch out for any phrase that might be interpreted as an admission of guilt, that I returned to my cell shivering all over. I had been severely ill and suffered from fevers before, but this "interrogation fever" was a thing apart. As a pathologist, I realized that it was the result of extreme stress that was wreaking havoc on my endocrine and nervous systems. It is generally believed that the effect of confinement in prison depends on its duration. My own experience of confinement in a special-regime prison shows that even a short sojourn there could have a devastating effect because of the strain one's forces of resistance are exposed to.

Back in my cell, I went over and over the details of each nighttime session. Did I let something drop that could be used against me or the others? And so a night of interrogation was followed by a day of self-interrogation, with not a minute's sleep to relieve the tension. But apparently I never did leave an opening for the investigator to use, since he said to me on several occasions: "Here you are protecting your cronies but, when the time comes, you'll be amazed to find out what they say about you." And he named some article of the Criminal Code according to which the accused was to be acquainted with the testimony of others being tried on the same charges. It may well have been that they did supply some compromising testimony against me, if we can judge by the passage from Miron Vovsi's testimony the investigator read out to me. Actually, when we were all released, Vovsi and Vinogradov themselves told me that they had admitted to all the crimes imputed to them. Vovsi said that they had even demanded an admission that he had spied for Germany. At that point he broke into tears: "What do you want of me? I have already admitted that I spied for England and America, isn't that enough? The Germans shot my whole family in Dvinsk, and you want me to say I was their spy!" "Stop this sniveling, you shit," the investigator bellowed, "go on and admit that you were a German spy!" So Vovsi signed that admission too. They succeeded in breaking Vinogradov's spirit as well. The most tragic aspect of these confessions was that the person admitted not only crimes he himself had supposedly committed, but also the existence of a criminal organization and collective criminal actions (article 58.11); so he was in fact exacerbating the lot of his "accessories." Having once owned up to imaginary crimes, the accused was led to cooperate with the investigation in exposing the crimes of the others. This happened to Vovsi and Vinogradov, and perhaps to other people as well.

Sophia Karpai, formerly a doctor at the Kremlin Hospital, told me in the summer of 1953 about her confrontation with Vovsi, Vinogradov, and Vasilenko in prison. To her face they asserted that she had executed their criminal orders to administer harmful treatments to her patients. She denied not only the fact of fulfilling such orders but also the fact of receiving them. The confrontation left her with the most dismal impression: had the professors gone mad? But they had not; it was simply a logical sequel to the admissions that had been forced out of them. Of course the confrontation was staged in the presence of the jailers, who were there for purposes of intimidation and who watched closely that the script elaborated by the investigation should be strictly adhered to.

So the people who had broken down became witnesses for the prosecution. Can we really condemn them for it? Fresh from prison, I had strong feelings on the subject and was not sure I would be able to overlook this "betrayal." But then I had a change of heart. I realized that one cannot demand heroism from everybody. People's powers of resistance vary greatly—from extreme tenacity to complete lack of physical courage. There are also different reactions to qualitatively different dangers. One and the same person may charge a tank, grenade in hand, and faint at the sight of a poised syringe. A friend of mine, a prominent scientist, told me frankly that, from what he knew about himself, if he had been arrested he would have broken down after half an hour's interrogation and complied with all demands made of him.

There was a deep general fear of torture, of which rumors were rife in the memorable purge years of 1937–1939. One despaired of being able to withstand it and was sure that, sooner or later, the required admissions would be extracted. Vinogradov told me that he had resolved from the beginning not to wait till they started torturing him but to admit all the charges, which included one of espionage for France and Great Britain.

We honor the courage and cherish the memory of those dauntless people who withstood torture by the Gestapo and did not betray their comrades, and we feel a mixture of pity and contempt for those who were broken. But those heroes were dying for a cause. What cause had the innocent doctors to die for? What good would a heroic death, in these besmirched circumstances, do the Soviet people? There was no moral stimulus for resistance to the methods "strictly forbidden by Soviet law" (a quotation from the government statement exonerating the doctors). On the other hand, if they toed the line, they could hope to avoid torture and a disgraceful death. And so, driven by that spectral hope (never justified, as experience showed), they slandered their friends and sometimes even members of their families.

This is how Miron Vovsi himself described his conduct in prison. Six years after the collapse of the Doctors' Plot, he developed sarcoma on his leg, which necessitated amputation (he died soon afterwards). I visited him on the second day after the operation and found him in an excited, euphoric state. "You cannot compare my present condition with what I felt *then*," he said. "Now I have merely lost a leg, but I am still a human being. But *there* I lost every vestige of humanity." That system deprived cultured, erudite, and, in normal conditions, decent people of their humanity. Imagine what mental suffering a person must have endured to regard such a calamity as the loss of a leg from cancer (and Vovsi certainly knew the grim outlook he faced) as a trifle compared with the tortured nightmare of the Doctors' Plot! Can one unequivocally condemn the victims of a system that succeeded in breaking even veteran revolutionaries, who had experienced tsarist prisons and penal servitude? A prisoner of Stalin's dungeons could rely only on determination to preserve a measure of human dignity, to withstand the savagery of the jailers, not to give in, not to betray. But for this, besides strength of character, one needed physical stamina, and in those days few medical professors, most of them elderly individuals, possessed it. Those who were broken need no justification, for justification is the handmaid of accusation. To understand is to forgive.

Despite my own stubbornness in prison, I am not at all sure that I would have been able to resist indefinitely. I recall the investigator's warning that little time was left for my admission of guilt and that, if I persisted in my denials, he would refuse to "work" with me and I would pass into other, apparently much harsher, hands. I could only interpret his words as a threat of torture. The day before, I had heard screams from the next room, the investigator's yells and foul curses. At times the screams faded into the kind of gruntlike groans one expects to hear from a person exhausted by torment. Was that hair-raising interlude staged especially for my benefit? When I was brought in for interrogation the next day, I was shaking all over from an apprehension of torture and from the inhuman effort of will I made to control it. The investigator noticed my condition and even asked solicitously if I needed a doctor. To this I said: "You intend to torture me, don't you? What has a doctor to do with it?" My investigator replied ironically: "So you expect to be put on the rack today?" I concluded that the screws were not to be applied just yet. Sometimes my nerves gave way and (no use denying it) I wept, but my determination to stand firm did not abandon me. I will never know if my resolve would have held out under the whole refined system of tortures used to extract confessions from the martyrs of Stalinism.

My investigator often rebuked me: "What kind of testimony is this? Like a bone thrown to a dog!" This was a figurative but fairly accurate description of the bits I let him have—information about the normal practice of a pathologist the likes of which he could obtain at any clinical or pathological conference in any hospital. Another reproach I often heard was: "You can't even be shown at an open trial." From these words I gathered that there would be a trial for "the murderers in white coats," at which they would confess to monstrous crimes, repent of them publicly, as so many unfortunates had done before them at open trials, and then be condemned to death notwithstanding. My jailers had obviously lost hope of reducing me to that abject condition. This reproach I perceived as the highest praise of my conduct, and I still take pride in it. I adhered to the end to the decision I had made with the support of my wife, my courageous and tender Sophia Yakovlevna—the decision not to give in.

I grew indifferent to such methods of interrogation as foul

language and abuse. I was equally impervious to the investigator's clumsy attempts to wound my pride when he said, for instance: "You're not even worthy of respect. When a person doesn't conceal that he is an enemy, one has to respect him. But you're just a dodger trying to evade responsibility for your crimes." I found these clumsy reproaches ludicrous. I prized the respect of worthy people, and what I tried to do in prison was to preserve it—and my self-respect as well. In my cell I recalled the words, "Prison is honor, not censure, for me," which the doomed Decembrist Ryleyev scratched on his tin bowl while confined in the Peter and Paul Fortress in 1825. Incidentally, had it occurred to me to scratch a motto on my bowl, the watchdogs in Lefortovo Prison would never have permitted it. When I once scratched a word on a piece of soap (a reminder of an argument I wanted to make to the investigator), a guard came in and confiscated the soap.

Another trick of the investigator was to ask an out-of-context question, such as: "Why did you say to Topchan, 'You can rest easy'?" I recalled the situation in which I had spoken these words over the telephone. Abram Topchan and I had a friend, Professor Sinai, who suffered from kidney stones, and in the spring of 1951 or 1952 an ambulance brought him to the urological clinic headed by Topchan. His condition was critical: both ureters were obstructed. All attempts to clear them had failed, and he developed symptoms of acute uremia. The only thing that could save him was an emergency operation, which Topchan performed; but it was too late and Sinai died. I performed the autopsy myself and saw that Sinai's condition was already hopeless when he was admitted to the clinic. Both sides of the pelvis were packed with gravel-like calculi, and there were irreversible changes in the kidneys themselves. No operation could have restored their function. (The techniques of kidney transplants or the artificial kidney had not yet been developed in the Soviet Union.) I still preserve in my files a photograph of Sinai's kidneys, which I took because of the extreme nature of the lesions.

141

Topchan was terribly upset by Sinai's death. He had a tender conscience and he took every death of a patient hard. And this particular patient had been a friend and an important man in the medical world. So Topchan was tortured by doubt—had he done everything that his duty as a physician and his experience as a surgeon demanded? He waited impatiently for the findings of the autopsy. That evening Topchan called me at home to seek reassurance. I gave him my objective verdict and said in conclusion: "You did everything that was humanly possible, and your conscience as a surgeon is clear; you can rest easy." I told the investigator all this, but he wouldn't part with his pet suspicions and droned on: "Why did you say, 'You can rest easy'? Was that a murder too?" Then an argument occurred to me that I thought he would appreciate: "But Sinai was a Jew too." He replied: "So what? Sometimes you must have found it necessary to kill Jews as well." Impeccable logic.

One of the more bewildering questions the investigator fired at me was: "What did you discuss at the house-warming party at E. G.'s?" I was flabbergasted—by the very fact of that name cropping up in connection with the Doctors' Plot. E. G. was a frail woman of about sixty who had recently had a stroke and whose interests were centered on her two adolescent grand-daughters. She was a prosector and pathologist at the hospital which was the base for some clinical departments, in particular those headed by Vovsi and Dunayevsky (a major urologist).

In the winter of 1951–52 E. G. held a house-warming party at her flat (in the same apartment building where I lived) to which she invited the Vovsis, the Dunayevskys, and the Rapoports. All of us accepted the invitation only to avoid offending her, since we were not among her close friends. Subsequently, all participants in this "assemblage" were arrested.

I had no clear recollections of the party, except that it was rather dull. It was all the more surprising to find the investigator treating it as an event of major importance. The very mention of E. G., a person inexpressibly distant from political concerns, seemed absurd. (Though, on second thought, why wasn't the arrest of professors Vovsi, Grinstein, and Feldman equally absurd?) At any rate, I told the investigator, "Surely this sickly old lady, who has no thought for anything but her granddaughters, had nothing to do with a political organization!" To this he growled: "A sickly old lady? Why, the bitch will croak here! You may survive, you're a strong man, but she'll croak for sure!" Inured as I had become to all kinds of absurdities, the idea of E. G. arrested as a political criminal seemed outlandish. To repeated questions about discussions that had taken place at the house-warming party, I said I couldn't recall anything of significance. We had toasted the hostess' health, admired the apartment, made all the usual compliments, and no political topic had been brought up. The investigator replied that they knew whose health we had drunk to and what compliments had been made. That was the last I heard about E. G. then. (When I got out of prison, one of the first questions I asked my wife was whether E. G. was back. My wife was puzzled and replied that she had never been arrested and was safely at home. So much for her "croaking" in prison. The Vovsis suspected that E. G. had been in the confidence of the MGB and that she had held the house-warming party on their orders.)

Another out-of-the-blue question was: "Do you know Professor Moshkovsky? What do you think of him?" I said, "He is a world-famous scientist, a loyal Soviet citizen, and a thoroughly decent man." "What? A loyal citizen? Why, he's a fucking whore, worse even than you!" This enlightened me to the fact that I was a metric unit of whoredom. On my release I was overjoyed to find the "fucking whore" hale, hearty, and unmolested, as was the "Jewish bourgeois nationalist" Topchan. Either the MGB had not got around to arresting them or the epithets were just more tricks aimed at confusing me.

Some questions seemed to have no meaning at all, such as: "How many times did you go to your dacha in 1952?" We spent most of that summer in Pärnu, Estonia, and did not go to the dacha at all. I did make a few trips there to attend to some household matters, but I attached no importance to them and it never occurred to me to count them. Still, by racking my memory, I was able to recall two such trips, but the investigator said I was lying, there had been three. Unable to remember the purpose of a third visit, I insisted there had only been two, and the stupid wrangling over this trifling matter continued for quite some time. At last I recalled that there had indeed been a third trip at the end of the summer, when I visited the Vovsis. This apparently was why the investigator attached special importance to that trip. Had I known beforehand that I would have to account for every movement, I might have kept a record. As it was, I often failed to answer questions of this type, and this was regarded as a deliberate denial of guilt.

I often wondered how the MGB obtained information about my trips to the dacha in the summer of 1952 and why they were interested in the matter. Surely they could not have shadowed my movements for a whole year. Now I had a pretty accurate idea of who their informant was. That summer, the Vovsis had rented a house that stood opposite mine and belonged to the very same E. G. When, years later, they told me they were convinced that E. G. had played a sinister role in the Doctors' Plot, I suddenly recalled a strange episode connected with her that had been an enigma to me for years.

It happened in the fall of 1952, while the Doctors' Plot was still being hatched. One day E. G. called me and asked my advice concerning a problem she had come up against. Mutual consultations were widely practiced among pathologists, so I saw nothing out of the ordinary in the request.

She told me about an autopsy she had performed on a young woman who died in the gynecological department of the hospital. The woman had been feeling well enough when suddenly she developed violent diarrhoea and other symptoms of severe intoxication and died within twenty-four hours. The doctors could not discover the cause of the intoxication, since all bacteriological tests (for dysentery and such) proved negative. The post-mortem, said E. G., had not shed any light either, so she asked my opinion. I thought that the clinical picture and the pathologist's findings were typical of arsenic poisoning, which is described in all textbooks of forensic medicine. Perhaps the possibility had simply not occurred to E. G. I always impressed on my students and subordinates that they must resort to forensic chemistry in all doubtful or suspicious cases. I advised E. G. to send a sample from the corpse she still had in her possession to be tested for arsenic (traces of it can be discovered chemically even in the hair). She said she would do so at once. Then she amplified my suggestion of the possibility of foul play with the following details, which smacked of a cheap detective novel.

During the patient's stay at the hospital, a nurse in the gynecological department had had an affair with the young woman's husband, an MGB colonel. This colonel, E. G. said, came to her to find out the results of the post-mortem and seemed to be more curious about the cause of his wife's death than grieved by his loss. He even said to her sarcastically: "You call yourself a pathologist, but you can't even establish the cause of death!" When I met E. G. again some time later, I inquired about the results of the chemical test and was amazed to hear that she had done nothing about it. This was incompatible with the civic duty of a pathologist (a professional crime, in fact), and I could only explain it by her reluctance to cross an MGB colonel. Fear of the MGB was not to be wondered at, although I thought it exaggerated in this case and, moreover, such timidity was not at all in her character. At the hospital she was known for her captiousness to attending doctors and her readiness to throw any errors they committed into their faces. Now here she was mumbling something incoherent and obviously reluctant to get to the root of the matter, at the cost of her professional integrity. I wondered how she worded her autopsy report on the nature of the disease and the cause of death. Had she invented a more or less feasible version, or had she written that the cause of death remained unclear (a pathologist is sometimes forced to admit failure)?

This situation tickled my curiosity for many years. I was

finally able to satisfy it, after E. G. died and a student of mine replaced her at the hospital. I asked him to have a look at the old autopsy records. I didn't know the name of the patient, and the record might have distorted the picture of the disease, but surely diarrhoea and vomiting could not be disguised as some gynecological ailment. Hard as my student tried, however, he was unable to discover the case E. G. had described. In fact there had been no deaths at all in the gynecological department during that period. So the incident remained a puzzle—for some thirty years. Then I had a flash of insight.

Since there had never been any such case, E. G. must have been probing me. There had been no young woman dying suddenly and in suspicious circumstances, no nurse who had an affair with the husband, an MGB colonel. The only real person, most probably, was the MGB colonel, who must have devised this rather primitive scheme for a "consultation" and rehearsed E. G.'s part with her. The only thing that was not quite clear was the purpose of the probe. Perhaps it was to ascertain my professional competence in light of the forthcoming Doctors' Plot, in which poisoning was to be the chief form of malpractice attributed to the culprits. Since the part assigned to me in the script of the plot was covering up the crimes of the killer doctors by falsifying post-mortem records, it may have occurred to the MGB to check my ability to establish—and consequently to conceal—a death by poisoning. (Recall the order given by an OGPU man to Abrikosov to look for traces of "Kazakov's potion" in performing the autopsy on Menzhinsky.) The schemes large and small elaborated by the MGB generally defied logic, but that was not considered a shortcoming. On the contrary, the less sense and logic, the more mystifying—and the more frightening—the accusation.

Some facts from my activities as a pathologist I simply could not recall. For instance, my investigator displayed an avid interest in the post-mortem examination of some infant performed by a pathologist from my department, Rosa Kogan. I could not remember the infant or what it had died of, but my investigator went into a hysterical frenzy, demanding that I should confess to my criminal role in the affair. He gasped, coughed, and all but vomited, tearing at the collar of his tunic and falling into such a state that my doctor's instincts were aroused and I rose to go to his aid. But he made a restraining gesture—what if I were to throttle him?—and recalling his solicitous inquiry at one of the interrogations, I in my turn asked if I should call a doctor. Today I cannot help smiling at the paradoxical situation—a manacled man fearing for the condition of his jailer.

The MGB's obsession with exposing conspiracies had infected my investigator. Indeed, if his bosses had uncovered a conspiracy of a truly global scope—the Doctors' Plot—why shouldn't he uncover his own little conspiracy, authored by him alone and corresponding to his rank and status? This would ensure immediate promotion. And so one day, apparently oblivious of the presence of one of the supposed conspirators (myself), he began outlining the conspiracy at the First Gradskaya Hospital that he expected to uncover in detail. He spoke fluently with animation, as if to an interested audience: "In the center is Topchan. The threads stretch from him to . . ." and he enumerated the Jewish doctors at the Gradskaya (some of them had already been arrested). He was for all the world like a young scientist reading a paper to an authoritative gathering on a major discovery he had made. My investigator did not even see me: before his mind's eye was an attentive and admiring audience consisting of MGB generals, and he, pointer in hand, was explaining to them the pattern of the conspiracy. He was in the grips of real creative ecstasy. The sight was so ludicrous that I burst out laughing. Caught by my mirth, he began laughing too, but pulled himself up at once and, his flight cut short, asked me sternly: "What are you laughing at?" "You looked so inspired painting the panorama of the conspiracy you yourself invented that I had to laugh." He resumed his professionally serious air and went on with the dull business of interrogation.

This was a very instructive little scene, which threw some

light on how conspiracies were fabricated within the walls of the MGB. Unbridled flights of crime-obsessed fantasy brought about the destruction of thousands of the best people. A man with an analytical cast of mind, I was fascinated to observe a conspiracy *statu nascendi*, in the process of birth.

So the grilling went on and on. I was supposed to invent my own crimes, a task for which I had neither the fantasy nor the desire. And apparently the time had not yet come for prompting. Perhaps the prompting was being postponed until my confrontation with some of the self-avowed terrorists, such as the meeting Sophia Karpai described to me. In the meantime my investigator had to be content with the "bones" I tossed him— admissions not of terrorist actions but of "terrorist utterances." There was my hearty "The devil take him!" addressed to Malenkov, which the informers had duly reported to the MGB. In the records the statement received the usual embellishment: "full of wild fury and brutal hatred . . ." When I asked the investigator why this particular utterance, which at worst was mere invective, was regarded as a wish for the abused person's death, my investigator answered: "But surely one must die before the devil can take him!" The devil himself was being recruited to serve the ends of the MGB. An atheist, as any party member was expected to be, the investigator apparently did not think that disbelief in the devil was also part of atheism. I denied that in speaking of the devil I had wished death to Malenkov, but the investigator merely droned on: "One must die before the devil can take him; that means you expressed a wish for Comrade Malenkov's death." At this point I thought about a scene in Swift's *Gulliver's Travels* where he describes the Academy of Lagado in Laputa (I have of course looked it up in order to quote accurately): "Another professor showed me a large paper of instructions for discovering plots and conspiracies against the government. He advised great statesmen to examine into the diet of all suspected persons; their times of eating; upon which side they lay in bed; with which hand they wiped their posteriors; to take a strict view of their excrements, and, from the colour, the odour, the taste, the consistence, the crudeness or maturity of digestion, form a judgment of their thoughts and designs." Finding the discourse "not altogether complete," Gulliver offers to "supply him with some additions."

> I told him that in the kingdom of Tribnia, by the natives called Langden, where I had sojourned some time in my travels, the bulk of the people consist in a manner wholly of discoverers, witnesses, informers, accusers, prosecutors, evidences, swearers, together with their several subservient and subaltern instruments, all under the colours and conduct of ministers of state and their deputies. The plots of that kingdom are usually the workmanship of those persons who desire to raise their own characters of profound politicians, to restore new vigour to a crazy administration, to stifle or divert general discontents, to fill their pockets with forefeitures, and raise or sink the opinion of public credit, as either shall best answer their private advantage. It is first agreed and settled among them, what suspected persons shall be accused of a plot; then, effectual care is taken to secure all their letters and papers, and put the criminals in chains. These papers are delivered to a set of artists, very dexterous in finding out the mysterious meanings of words, syllables, and letters. For instance, they can discover a close-stool to signify a privy council; . . . a broom, a revolution; . . . an empty tun, a general; a running sore, the administration.

Across the centuries Jonathan Swift, that man of genius, uncovered the secret workings of security bodies in Stalin's Laputa. He might have painted his picture from nature, so great was the resemblance between the MGB system and that of Tribnia.

As I recalled these pages from *Gulliver's Travels* in my cell, I drew from them that charge of humor I needed so much to fight off the devilry of the interrogation. To keep my sanity, I had to keep faith in "that old common arbitrator, Time," as Shakespeare put it, to hold on to the memory of the real world outside the walls of that madhouse, the world in which I had lived for more than fifty years. The hardest hours were between lunch and supper, when dusk fell and I sat, manacled, in the oppressive silence of the prison, awaiting yet another interrogation, with all its stupidities and the desperate need to parry them. I had to find an escape—and I found it.

In my mind I began to compose a course of general pathology, a book I had planned to write for a long time. I had been collecting material for the book for years. And so, sitting on my bed, I delivered to an imaginary audience lectures that comprised a systematic course. I got quite carried away, for it was interesting, creative work. It is a pity I was unable to write down many ideas that occurred to me then, since some of them are irretrievably lost. Even in a Gestapo prison, Julius Fučik was able to write his "Reporting with a Noose around My Neck," but a prisoner in Stalin's dungeons was not allowed even that much liberty. True, Lina Stern apparently did some work in Lubyanka Prison, for she brought back a manuscript on histohematic barriers. But this was permitted only after the investigation was over and the sentence passed—exile to Jambul, which was in fact the mildest punishment possible, seeing that all the others accused at that trial were shot. In my case, the firing squad was a certainty if Stalin had not died when he did.

My interrogation was obviously approaching the culmination point. Once (at the end of February or early March) the investigator again warned me that not only the days but even the hours for a voluntary admission of guilt were running out. He said in this connection, "I am not your enemy," but immediately corrected himself: "Of course I'm not your friend either. But I want you to know that Stalin himself is following the course of the investigation, and he is displeased with your conduct. Keep this in mind—you'll have only yourself to blame." I didn't give much credence to his words about Stalin, since I was hardly important enough to attract Stalin's interest. But at the Twentieth Party Congress, in Khrushchev's report on the personality cult, Stalin's interest in the investigation of the Doctors' Plot was confirmed, and it may well be that he did take notice of those who denied their crimes and recommended that strong measures be applied. But at the time I merely thought that the investigator was trying to intimidate me.

Then one evening my interrogator said he needed me as an expert. Would I answer some professional questions, such as what was Cheyne-Stokes respiration? I explained that it was a kind of spasmodic, interrupted breathing. "When does it occur?" I answered that it occurred physiologically in newborn infants and appeared in adults when severe lesions of the respiratory centers in the brain were present—as in brain tumors, cerebral hemorrhages, uremia, or severe arteriosclerosis. "How can Cheyne-Stokes respiration be controlled?" One had to control its causes, not the respiration as such. "Can a person who has Cheyne-Stokes respiration recover?" It was a grave symptom, often attending the agonies of death, and in the majority of cases death was inevitable. He wrote down my answers with seeming imperturbability. I thought all this had to do with some foul play attributed to the doctors who had been arrested. Then the investigator went on to ask which major specialist I would recommend to attend a patient in such critical condition. When I replied that I had no idea which major specialists were still free, that put him in a quandary. A prisoner in a special-regime prison could on no account be given information about events beyond its walls. So he said: "Just name whoever you think is the best." I replied:

Vinogradov is an excellent doctor, but he's in prison. Vovsi is also a splendid specialist, but you have him too. Vasilenko has great experience in such diseases, but he is incarcerated as well. Etinger is a brilliant diagnostician, but you know where he is. Both Kogans are efficient doctors, but one is long dead and the other is in prison. If you want a neuropathologist, I regard Grinstein as the best clinical neuropathologist, but he's in your hands too. Among the otolaryngologists, I could recommend Preobrazhensky or Feldman, but they're both locked up.

In short, I enumerated all the major specialists who, as I knew, were in prison and suggested that he should name some who were not. After some thought he named four persons. I said that not one of them (although two were regarded as luminaries of Soviet medical science) measured up to the specialists I had mentioned. The investigator was greatly surprised and began arguing with me, saying that one of the four was a member of the Academy of Medical Sciences. To this I replied that he had asked me to recommend a good doctor, not an academician, and that these two roles were not identical. Only one of the four, in my opinion, was a competent physician, but on a much lower level than the men in prison.

When I was released from prison and read the newspapers for February and March of 1953, I realized that the investigator had been picking my brain in connection with Stalin's illness. I learned that Miron Vovsi and Eliazar Gelstein had also been consulted and that their testimonials had been very similar to mine. As I now recall that session, I feel that Stalin's associates wanted to find out if he could recover, if the doctors attending him might still get him back on his feet. My verdict must have reassured them, and it was soon borne out by events: Stalin died on March 5. However, in my solitary cell in Lefortovo, I had no inkling of this significant event and no means of knowing that the timely death was going to save my life and the lives of my colleagues, and would mark a radical change in the social and political climate of the Soviet Union.

After this "consultation," nothing changed: the same handcuffs and the same nightly interrogations, even though there was a perceptible lessening of pressure. The investigator grew lazy, was less emphatic in his questions, and often went out, leaving me in the charge of a guard, who kept dozing off as he sat on a settee and jumping awake with a guilty smile. I also used these absences for snatching naps. Generally, though the drumming continued, it lost its urgency.

On March 9 (I remember this date well) I was suddenly summoned for an interrogation in the daytime and brought to a different room. There I saw my investigator and a man in the uniform of a colonel. The colonel's appearance struck me as unusually repulsive and vicious. A puny man, he had the face of some small carnivore, a rat or a polecat, breathing hatred for all men. "God," I thought, "this bodes no good." The colonel conducted the interrogation, while my curator played up to him obsequiously. The colonel's questions were liberally seasoned with obscenities. My interrogator also used to swear at me now and then but never so ferociously, and I occasionally reciprocated, to show that I had also been introduced to the "elegance of leisurely spoken Russian" (Balmont's line) and that I had a good command of that particular idiom, Jewish bourgeois nationalist though I might be. But mostly I did it to indicate that his language did not ruffle me in the least. In my conversation with the colonel, little reference was made to terrorist activities. I tried to explain that any doctor is bound to make an error now and then, that these errors are openly discussed at clinical and anatomical conferences with no legal intercession required, except in those rare cases when a death was due to criminal negligence. I said I had known major doctors, including Bakulev, who had committed errors and frankly admitted them, sometimes even prior to an autopsy. My savage opponent growled: "We shall get around to Bakulev!" I had had occasion to discuss the possibility of errors with my investigator. When he declared once that the MGB never made mistakes (in reply to my assertion that my arrest had been a mistake), I told him that both doctors and investigators made mistakes, though the rate of mortality in the latter case was incomparably higher. When I said something like this to the colonel, he burst into a stream of obscenities, whereas my investigator had confined himself to reasserting the MGB's infallibility.

153

For some reason, the colonel's interrogation centered on my attitude to Georgy Malenkov. My dossier contained information about my use of such epithets as "son of a bitch" and "stinker" in reference to the deputy premier. I did not deny it, for I might very well have used those words. The colonel raved on about my ingratitude, for had not Malenkov done a lot for our victory over Nazi Germany? On this I made no comment. Then followed an exchange that I can quote almost verbatim, so strong an impression did it make on me.

"Did he drag a lot of Jews into his department?" the colonel asked my investigator.

"No, he didn't have time," was the obsequious answer.

"Why didn't I have time?" I interposed. "I worked there for many years."

"Give me the names of your staff," the colonel demanded.

"Arkhangelskaya."

"Name and patronymic!"

"Nadezhda Vasilyevna."

"A Jewess!" cried the colonel.

"What, Arkhangelskaya a Jewess?"

"Yes, so she is."

I felt dazed. I recalled that Arkhangelskaya did have a slightly aquiline nose. Could the MGB be right?

"Next!" demanded the colonel.

"Berezovskaya."

"Name and patronymic!"

"Elena Konstantinovna."

"A Jewess!"

Again I was confused. Berezovskaya's husband was a Jew—could she have been concealing her own nationality from me?

"Next!"

"G."

"Name and patronymic!"

"Cleopatra Alexeyevna."

"A Jewess!"

At this point I realized that some kind of absurd farce was being enacted and stopped taking the colonel's verdicts seriously.

"Who else?" demanded the colonel.

"Baranov."

"Name and patronymic!"

"Alexei Ivanovich."

"A Jew!"

"If Baranov is a Jew, then I have only one Russian on my staff—Rachel Pinkhusovna Kogan."

"Do you think I'm going to listen to your fucking wise-cracks?" roared the colonel. "You betrayed us when we suggested that you work for us, and now you think you can poke fun at us?"

The last thing I could afford was to poke fun at my tormentors. I had simply been unable to contain myself. The meaning of that farce will forever remain a mystery to me.

On the other hand, the shifting of the stress from terrorism to insulting Malenkov obviously had a meaning—which only became clear later when the alignment of forces was revealed at the Twentieth Congress in 1956. But, in any event, I was able to gather that the chief charge now was denigrating Malenkov—which, by the standards of the time, was also a state crime. All the more surprising, therefore, was the conclusion of my meeting with the colonel: he ordered my handcuffs removed.

I racked my brain about the meaning of this ludicrous scene. Why had the colonel honored me with a talk in the middle of the day? Just to make sure of my attitude to Malenkov? My investigator knew all about it and could easily have composed a proper protocol including the slurs "son of a bitch" and "stinker."

Immured in Lefortovo, I was ignorant of things the colonel knew. He knew that Stalin was being buried that very day, that the threads of the Doctors' Plot had begun unwinding, that their medical experts were already taking back their incriminating testimonies. He knew that Malenkov was at the head of the new government and, in slavish zeal, must have decided to try and get on his good side. The Doctors' Plot was going up in smoke, and he, one of its promoters, was in danger of losing face. So why not try and use one of the "terrorists" to cook up another dish? Perhaps the new head of government might relish it? Well, nothing came of it. It seemed the taste for such spicy dishes went out along with the chef.

Freed of the handcuffs and, with them, the other "restrictive measures," as soon as I returned to my cell I demanded to be shaved. The shaving was performed by one of the guards, with a safety razor. Then the pushcart arrived with some decent edibles—sausages, butter, biscuits. I was again living the normal life of a special-regime prisoner, including periodic walks in the concrete pen. I accepted all these boons without quite understanding how I had earned them. Why the colonel, after all but annihilating me, had suddenly had a change of heart and amnestied me was a mystery.

At the next session my investigator informed me that the investigation would go on, but his heart was obviously no longer in it. We had some chats on extraneous subjects, during one of which I explained the biological and philosophical foundations of my optimism. He seemed deflated, more and more often went off during the night, returning toward morning and hastily scrawling some semblance of an examination form half a page long. I was quite bored with signing these dull, uninspired compositions: no more "wild fury" or "brutal hatred."

One night the investigator produced several typewritten pages from my thick file and began reading them aloud, without explaining where they had come from and pretending that they had nothing to do with me. From time to time, he darted a sly glance at me—had I recognized it? I certainly had. It was the autopsy report on a young woman who had died in Feugel's clinic—the very case over which I disagreed with Cleopatra G., who performed the autopsy and came up with postpuerperal sepsis. So the report *had* made its way into the dossier as evidence of my connivance in the criminal acts of Jewish doctors. Joining in the game, I pretended I had never seen the report and made comments as he read on. The autopsy report had a supplement—the summary of a histological examination of some organs of the deceased (primarily the uterus). This demonstrated ignorance in both formulation and interpretation of the histological picture, which was twisted to prove sepsis. Such a document could never fool a professional. I analyzed the report in detail, trying to demonstrate its author's incompetence in terms the investigator would understand, and suggested that the examination must have been the work not of a professional pathologist but of some police doctor, little versed in pathology and more at home in cases of defloration in rape or injuries sustained in drunken brawls. But the investigator insisted that the histological examination had been done by an eminent pathologist. At the same time, his whole demeanor suggested that he did not put much faith in the pathologist's eminence, and he even voiced a suspicion that the aim had been to misdirect the investigation for some shady personal end. This was something new—the investigator expressing contempt for a report previously regarded as proof against me.

For many years I tried to guess the identity of that "eminent pathologist," an expert for the MGB. Finally my suspicions settled on a major pathologist who is dead now. Although I never voiced my suspicions (and generally did not discuss the matter with anybody), in my thoughts I have asked that man's forgiveness over and over again, because I was wrong. I learned later who the real author of that pseudo-scientific denunciation was, from the histologist Grigory Roskin. He once asked me if I knew who had played the most perfidious role in my case. When I said no, he told me he had irrefutable proof that it had been Boris Mogilnitsky. Mogilnitsky had angled, quite persistently, for the post of expert in the Doctors' Plot, and on his own initiative sent to the MGB distorted materials intended to compromise me. Then everything fell into place.

The only thing that still surprised me was why I had not

guessed earlier. The autopsy report and supplement could only have come from G.—her role in the affair seemed quite obvious. But I believed she had sent not only the autopsy report but also organ samples for a histological examination to the MGB so they could be done by an MGB expert. Apparently she had done nothing of the kind but asked Professor Mogilnitsky to examine the samples (perhaps in order to get an expert opinion on my conclusion), and it was Mogilnitsky who forwarded his falsified histological report to the MGB. I always had good reason to regard Mogilnitsky as a scoundrel in general and an ignoramus as far as pathology was concerned, and now my opinion was well confirmed. During my interrogation I had sometimes wondered how the investigator knew about my relations with G. and her relations with Mogilnitsky. Once when I permitted myself a hostile if restrained comment on the person of G., my investigator asked me why I disliked G. and himself suggested the explanation: "Is it because she works for Mogilnitsky?"

Shortly before her death (by suicide), G. swore tearfully to me that she had not denounced me to the MGB. I did not believe her then, but now I am inclined to think that she might have not known about the subsequent fate of the autopsy materials she forwarded to Mogilnitsky. I have devoted so much space to this personal episode because it throws light on the general climate in the medical world fostered by Stalin's regime.

I knew it was all winding down, but I cannot say that I awaited the end of the investigation with impatience. At best, I could count on concentration camp and exile. There was just a flicker of hope that time would work a change in my fate. I was fortunate—the change came much earlier than I expected.

– 8 –

Refutations

ON MARCH 14 a prison guard entered my cell as usual, but instead of taking me to another interrogation, he led me downstairs to the room where I had been welcomed upon my arrival at Lefortovo. I was again met by the same attractive woman doctor, who went through the same ritual of body search, including inspection of my anus. When this was over, I was put into the limousine I already knew so well, and after a rather long ride I found myself again in the inner yard of the Lubyanka building and then, through a door, in a box. The latter architectural detail is worth special mention, and I hope it will remain of purely literary interest to the reader. The box is a tiny room, the size of an ordinary wardrobe, into which the prisoner is pushed each time there is a danger of his running into someone he should not see, such as another prisoner on his way along the endless prison corridors (all of which contain rows of boxes). The guards leading the prisoners signal their approach by snapping their fingers (in Lefortovo) or tapping a key on a buckle (in Lubyanka). Thus, by this signal alone, the prisoner can tell which prison he is in even if he is blindfolded. This snapping or tapping is often the only sound in the gravelike silence of the strict-regime prison.

The box in which I was locked this time was a bit larger than a wardrobe and had a bench inside. Here I sat in a stupor with no thoughts about what was in store for me. A good thing, since my prospects were anything but cheerful. I heard a telephone ring outside and my name pronounced by the officer on duty. The door opened and I was taken by elevator up to some higher floor. After winding through another labyrinth of corridors with doors on both sides, I was led into one of the rooms where a stocky gray-haired general sat at his desk facing the door. I immediately recognized him: he had been present at one of my interrogations but hadn't said a word. The chair to the left of the desk was occupied by the colonel with the face of a polecat, whom I knew much better: it was he who had interrogated me on March 9, insisting that all my colleagues were Jews. In a darkish corner (I didn't catch sight of him at once) sat my investigator. The general greeted me in an unexpectedly cordial manner, like a health-spa doctor greeting a newly arrived patient: "Good afternoon, Yakov Lvovich!" The general did not introduce himself (and I still don't know his name), so I could not return the cordiality and answered shortly: "Good afternoon." I was not so much encouraged as surprised by the warmth of his tone. In such an office, a greeting like that might be a mocking prelude to something terrible, a cat-and-mouse game. This is why the general's attentive and, as it seemed to me, benevolent look as well as the remark he addressed to the colonel—"Why is the professor such a sorry sight?"—made me apprehensive. I was astonished to hear myself called "professor" in this of all places, where I was classified as "an enemy of the people." And I was amazed to hear the note of reproach addressed to the colonel, unless it was meant as a taunt.

The "professor" did not look like one at all: closely cropped, unshaven, a long nose on a shrunken face, dressed in a prison robe with no buttons, a crumpled jacket also without buttons, loose trousers barely held up by one remaining button. In my cell, when I had a chance to catch my reflection in the water-filled basin, my only mirror, I could see I was no picture of male beauty. My anger overwhelmed me now: "Why, I must look terrifying, I presume, as befits a Jewish terrorist!" The general responded to the bitter outburst with the following words, which I quote almost verbatim: "Yakov Lvovich, please forget what happened at the interrogation. You know, anything can happen during an investigation [this sounded like an apology of sorts]. Can you tell me in all frankness what really happened? Don't fear that you'll be made to suffer for your words. I give you my word of honor that nothing you say will have any consequences." I answered without a moment's hesitation:

Nothing whatsoever happened. The doctors are all honest Soviet citizens, all devoted to the Soviet homeland and to their chosen profession. The one thing that really happened was national discrimination among the professors, inspired and fanned by a few prejudiced scoundrels, some of them card-bearing party members. They are mainly responsible for the discrimination at my institute and for the persecution of Jewish professors. The latter were driven either to voice their protest or to fall into a deep depression—particularly when they were sacked, one by one, on different pretexts.

"But were they all honest Soviet citizens?!" the general half queried, half asserted. To this I exclaimed: "Of course! They are excellent teachers and talented scientists. They have educated thousands upon thousands of doctors, and it is largely thanks to their efforts that Moscow's Second Medical Institute enjoys the reputation of being the best in the Soviet Union." I went on to quote numerous facts of discrimination practiced against Jews, including the charge of "Jewish bourgeois nationalism." Then the general asked me if I knew Miron Vovsi. I explained that I had known Vovsi for a good many years and, for the life of me, could not see him as a political figure. He was never interested in politics because of certain traits of character. I said I knew of Vovsi's present plight and that he had admitted to being involved in terrorism and espionage, but still this admission seemed completely incompatible with my image of him (at this point the general and the colonel exchanged meaningful glances).

I went on: the statement of January 13, 1953, alleging that Vovsi was the leader of an anti-Soviet terrorist organization, had come as a complete surprise to me. It was the last thing one would expect from a man like him. Besides, during World War II, Vovsi had served as chief internist of the Red Army and coped with his duties admirably. The very fact that he was entrusted with a task of state importance suggested that he had been thoroughly checked. So the unspeakable accusations against him had come like a bolt from the blue. In all my years with Vovsi, I could not recall his saying a single thing on a political subject. I was the one who did most of the talking. For instance, I remember telling him about the disturbing situation at the Institute of Morphology, and he just listened. Now it appeared that, all this time, he had been the leader of an anti-Soviet organization of which I was also a member! I had learned at the prison that another member of this organization was supposed to be Efim Vovsi, brother of the actor Mikhoels and Miron's cousin. But I was barely acquainted with Efim. I had seen him several times at the neighboring dacha that Miron was renting. Actually I did not so much see as hear him: he loved singing, to the great distress of his neighbors, for he was a poor singer. Imagine our being members of the same criminal organization, of which neither of us had an inkling before being arrested . . .

The general was also interested in my work as a pathologist, in light of the crimes I was charged with. I described the relationship between pathologist and clinician, in about the same terms as I have done in this book, stressing the importance of the pathologist's tact and good will toward the clinician. I personally never assumed the attitude of a judge and impressed on my students and staff that they should never do so either. They should put themselves in the shoes of the attending doctor dealing with a difficult case. The task of the pathologist is not to pass judgment but to reveal the nature of the disease and the essence of the error, if one has been made in treatment. During my long career I had discovered quite a few serious errors in the work of major clinicians, even those of world renown. If I had charged them with criminal intent each time, I would have showered investigative bodies with denunciations. I recalled a certain Dr. R., Bakulev's assistant and subsequently a professor at a provincial university, who came to me to confess a serious surgical error he had made that he expected would lead to a fatal outcome (which was indeed the case). Was I supposed to bring charges against him? Similar errors were committed by celebrated surgeons, even at the peak of their careers. No, we discussed R.'s error at a doctors' conference in the presence of his supervisor, Bakulev, so that he as well as his colleagues could draw a lesson from it. One thing I always insisted on was painstaking care in drawing up post-mortem reports, which had to contain every single detail and every defect in the treatment revealed by the autopsy, because this information has enormous instructive importance. A post-mortem report is an official document. I never hushed up doctors' errors, but neither did I use them to intimidate others. And now all that had been twisted to make it appear as if I had been covering up terrorist murders . . .

That was how I put it all to the general, who listened to my story with great attention and, it seemed to me, understanding. I was frank, for I had nothing to lose. I expounded my professional and political principles and, judging by the expression on the general's face, he sympathized with my sentiments. The colonel, on the other hand, showed complete lack of interest and hostile indifference. I didn't really pay attention to him. I sensed that he didn't count here, since he had been reproached for my "sorry appearance." The subject of Israel was touched upon in passing, but it was of little relevance in the general context of this discussion. Neither the general nor I dwelled at any length upon Israel, since the subject was not as urgent then as it became later. I remember saying that I sympathized with the country's struggle for independence.

I can't remember how long my passionate speech lasted. It added nothing new to what I had said during my interrogations. This time they did not embellish the record with their favorite metaphors, "with venomous hate" or "with savage hatred toward the Soviet system." I spoke with great feeling, for I had to defend not only myself but the whole of Soviet medicine, Soviet science, Soviet Jews, and common sense in general. In my oration I rejected vigorously the accusations of terrorism against the medical professors. The accusations were absurd, even though the accused had pleaded guilty (as the general had aptly said, "Anything can happen during an investigation"). I based my conviction on a long and close association with all the accused: Vinogradov, Vovsi, Vasilenko, Zelenin, Etinger, the Kogan brothers, Grinstein, Preobrazhensky, and others, none of whom was capable of evil intent toward their patients. I could admit, theoretically, that a person might go mad and commit a horrible crime in a fit of frenzy, but the idea of group madness going on for such a long time could occur only to a lunatic. I made more than good use of the general's offer to speak frankly and spoke my mind in the harshest language. Again, I had nothing to lose.

Having heard me out, the general asked me whether any of us had considered the possibility of emigrating to the United States. I answered curtly: "I gave my all to my country. My daughters are Young Communist members, and I am a Communist. I have never considered emigrating to America." The general concluded our conversation with a meaningful remark addressed to the colonel: "The matter seems to be clear." To which the colonel answered: "Yes, sir!"

"Yakov Lvovich, we shall keep you here for as long as it takes you to put down in writing everything you've just told us here," said the general and left. As I was led out of the room the colonel said: "So much for handcuffs." This may have been some kind of apology, for I suspect I had been handcuffed on the colonel's orders. Pointedly looking down at him, not just because he was seated but because I wanted to show him how much I despised him, I answered: "Everyone to his own devices. I have my microscope and you have your handcuffs.

Only you haven't accomplished anything by your methods." With these words I left the room in great emotional turmoil, sensing rather than understanding that something important had happened. A ray of common sense had burst into the collective nightmare in which we had been living.

I remember subsequent events as in a dream. I lost track of time. I remember being taken to a spacious windowless room with a low ceiling. There was a bed, a table laid in the usual prison manner, and a chair. I had the impression that it was not a regular cell but a basement room hastily furnished to receive a prisoner for a short spell. On the table were several sheets of paper, a pen, and an inkwell. I was too excited and exhausted to start writing immediately. I knocked on the door to summon the guard and told him that I was in need of some rest before I could start writing my statement. I asked permission to sleep first, although by now it was daytime. The guard left and came back with permission for me to take a nap. But still I was too excited to sleep. I needed some outlet, so I sat down and started writing one page after another (I can imagine what trouble they had deciphering those scribbles made worse by nervous excitement). I used up all the paper: they had not counted on this fit of graphomania. My request for more paper annoyed my jailers, who were used to laconic reports and verdicts.

Later I could not for the life of me remember what I had filled eighteen pages with. It was no doubt a repetition of what I had poured out to the general. I do remember describing the activities of several people at my institute, calling them scoundrels and antisemites. I did write about the general atmosphere in the strict-regime prison, about being deprived of sleep for days on end, about the handcuffs that cut into my wrists, about libelous evidence being obtained under pressure and the resistance I had put up. I mentioned the embellishments with which quite innocent words and episodes were adorned in the interrogation records. I handed in my statement to the prison guard and never knew what happened to it. I only wish I could have a look today at that violent attack on the establishment that kept me prisoner.

I expected to be released immediately after I had finished writing. So you can imagine my disappointment and anxiety when, the next day, I was pushed into a Black Raven and transported back to my old cell in Lefortovo Prison. Was the whole incident just more of the playacting that the MGB people were so good at? Their love of cat-and-mouse was well known, with the unavoidable outcome for the mouse and the great creative variety that the cats could bring to the game. Had I been a gullible mouse? Only an inveterate skeptic could have believed, in those circumstances, that he had been fooled, and skepticism was not in my nature. For all my anxiety, I did trust in the genuineness of the events the day before.

Although I was worried, there were obvious changes in the climate at Lefortovo. First of all, the interrogations stopped. The first few nights I was waiting for them at the usual hour; the signal to go to bed sounded, but no one came to take me to an interrogation. It reminded me of the neurotic man who waits every night for his neighbor to take off his boots with the usual clatter before he can go to sleep. Now allowed to sleep, I was unable to. Logic told me that the summons to Lubyanka had not been accidental and was bound to have some consequences. But I had no means of finding out exactly what had happened, what had caused this dramatic change or whether any change had really taken place. I was still being detained in the same prison, in strict isolation from the rest of the world. Now I did not even have contact with the prison guards, who used to visit me at least three times a day to put on and take off my hand-cuffs. Now I had no contact with my investigator, who had disappeared; there were no more summons to his office. I racked my brain, trying to think of some way to obtain information about what was going on, if only an inkling, so that I could fill in the rest. Then I thought of a trick: I banged on the door of my cell to call the guard. I told him I needed my glasses. Only my investigator could issue permission for anything concerning my person, as he himself had informed me at our first meeting. The guard said he would communicate my request. To be on the safe side, I also said I had important information for the ears of my investigator alone.

I expected to be summoned that same evening, but no summons came. Only the next day did the guard come to take me to the investigator's office. My curator was in his overcoat, as if he had just dropped in for a minute. He was sorting out papers on his desk, tearing some of them to shreds and stuffing them into the wastepaper basket. He met me with a hostile look, declaring that it was I who wanted to see him, not vice versa, and I should bear that in mind. He was clearly no longer interested in me and no longer in charge of my case. The way he was cleaning his desk of accumulated papers was some evidence of change. He asked me what I wanted of him. The tables were turned and it was not he who wanted something—another significant detail. I told him of my nervous condition, verging on psychosis, because I could not understand what was going on, why the investigation had been stopped and what that meant for me. To this day I gratefully recall his answer. I was not mistaken in him: he did have some humanity and intelligence. He reproached me for presenting him in the wrong light in my report, so I deduced that he had read it and had been censured for distorting my evidence. This meant they believed me, which was like a breath of fresh air. Then he resumed his usual genial manner and said that I would soon be summoned to the Lubyanka office and that all would end well. I was overcome with gratitude for this piece of news. (He also issued permission for the warden to give me my glasses.)

I returned to my cell in agitation. Could all this be true? My heart was nearly bursting with anticipation, with the awareness that I was no longer grist for the MGB's maniacal mill and would soon be a normal person again. That was enough to take away sleep. As I tried to picture the various scenarios awaiting me, little did I think that it might be complete rehabilitation. Certainly I was guilty of cursing Malenkov (thank God not

Stalin himself, for that would have meant capital punishment) and for asserting the existence of antisemitism in the Soviet Union. So, in Stalinist terms, the best I could hope for was exile (for some reason, I hoped it would be to Guryev). One thought I remember distinctly: if they offered me a choice of deportation from the country or internal exile, I would choose exile without hesitation; then I could return to normal life as soon as things took a turn for the better. And one day they would, I had no doubt—if only I survived to see it. I did not want to live the life of an emigré, for I had heard much about the hard lot of postrevolutionary emigrés. My train of thought was typical of the Stalinist era: an innocent victim choosing a punishment for himself for a crime he never committed. Only solitary confinement could give rise to such fantasies.

After the tension of my nightly verbal duels with the investigator, after the expectation of a tragic outcome, after the excitement of the recent meeting at the Lubyanka office followed by return to the same cell and encouraging information from my investigator, I was now living the undisturbed life of a prisoner in solitary confinement. No one took any interest in me. I was alone with my thoughts, which were interrupted a few times a day by daily prison events: reveille, breakfast, lunch, supper, and the signal for bedtime. I filled the long hours of each day by reciting poems from memory or recalling books I'd read. Sometimes I played whole pieces of music in my mind, those I could resurrect in my memory.

One day I heard the sound of a pushcart I had never heard before. It stopped at the door of my cell; the hatch through which my meals were served opened, and a hand thrust in two books. It was the prison library supplying the prisoners with "mental pabulum." I threw myself greedily on those rations for which my mind had been starving and which henceforth were regularly doled out. The books were quite good for the most part: Russian classics and some Soviet books I hadn't read before. I could not help noting the unusual assortment, testifying to the librarians' unexpected literary taste, and the good printing quality of the prison tomes. It was also surprising that I was never offered any political books, which one would have expected for the reform of Lefortovo's political prisoners. In those days, even outside prison, volumes of political propaganda were nauseatingly conspicuous. Without a doubt, if books could speak not only the language of their authors but also that of their former owners, they would have much to tell about themselves and of the sorrowful path that had brought them to Lefortovo Prison, in accord with the established procedure of property confiscation.

Thus it happened that Lefortovo gave me a chance to fill in the gaps in my literary education. I remember particularly vividly how I was introduced to the Polish writer Maria Konopnicka. I had never before read anything by this remarkable poet and prose writer. I virtually fell in love with her and her work. She seemed to me an attractive woman of much the same cast of mind as my own, whose views I could identify with. I learned some of her poems by heart and even set some of them to music as hymns or love songs (I would never have dared to perform my creations aloud, even in solitary confinement). When I was released from prison, almost the first thing I did was to rush to a secondhand bookshop and buy an anthology of her work, which took a place of honor in my bookcase. Naturally prisoners did not have the right to choose which books to read. We had to take what we were given. I remember asking the librarian if he could exchange the book he was giving me because I had read it before. He asked me: "Where have you read it, here?" "No, at home." "Then read it here now," he snapped. For him a book was just another type of ration. Quite possibly, both our food and our intellectual rations were distributed by one and the same person.

The barred window under the ceiling of my cell faced east, and early in the morning a sun ray lit the ceiling, moving along its perimeter to die down in the opposite corner. It was indeed a ray of light in the realm of darkness.

All this went on until March 21, when I was again led downstairs and a Black Raven took me to Lubyanka. Again I was led along countless corridors lined with boxes, into which I was pushed from time to time. Eventually I was brought to a big room where ten or twelve people in civilian clothes were sitting, either behind desks or in armchairs. In the center of this group sat a colonel wearing a badge that read "Honored Cheka Officer." He conducted the proceedings, which were in the nature of a free exchange of opinions between the accused and all those present, with no time limits imposed. Colonel Kozlov (if I remember the name correctly) opened the proceedings with the request that I tell them everything concerning my arrest and the investigation.

As a Jewish bourgeois nationalist, I concentrated, as would be expected, on the accursed "Jewish question." I was quite outspoken in expressing my indignation as a witness and object of discrimination against Jews. I mentioned the numerous cases when talented people were refused jobs at scientific research institutes. I told them in particular how my most promising student, Tatyana Ivanovskaya (née Marukhes, now a noted professor who holds the chair of pathology at the Second Medical Institute), was finally allowed to join the staff of my laboratory only as a junior research fellow. Her father was a baptized Jew who had married a Christian. In tsarist Russia, intermarriage between Jews and Christians was prohibited, so Jews had to convert if they wanted to marry a Christian. The head of the personnel department, Zilov, noted her maiden name, betraying her half-Jewish origin, and refused her the job. It so happened that not only had Ivanovskaya been christened at birth but that she had preserved the baptism certificate issued by the priest. When I learned about this interesting detail, I urged her to show the certificate to Zilov and convey my request that it be included in her file. Despite her reluctance, Ivanovskaya did as I told her, and the next day she got the job, although Zilov feigned indifference to her piece of evidence.

I gave many more examples of discrimination against Jews in employment at research centers and in personnel reductions. As an internationalist and a Communist, I could never reconcile

170

myself to this. The subject of discrimination caused a lively debate, and since those present were unable to disprove the facts I was quoting, the colonel asked a general question: "Do you think it normal that at some research institutes 50 percent of personnel are Jews?" I answered: "If you asked me whether I thought it normal that at some research institutes 50 percent of personnel are idiots and nincompoops, I would agree it was not normal. In a scientist only his value to science matters—not his nationality." I went on to say that before wages were raised at the research centers, no one bothered to count the number of Jews working there. As for myself, after graduation I had chosen a low-paying theoretical discipline, and at that time no one was interested in my nationality, except for some traditionally antisemitic prerevolutionary professors.

I also told them the story of the plan to publish a manual on histological diagnosis of tumors, when Shabad and I had been crossed off the list of authors. I spoke with particular passion about the traumatic experiences that Jewish boys and girls were subjected to at the entrance examinations to colleges and universities, when examiners deliberately failed them in a manner insulting to their dignity. I also told them how my young daughter was accused of servility toward the United States and of antipatriotism by her history teacher. My interlocutors urged me to ignore "that fool."

In fact, they tried to convince me that discrimination was not the result of some national policy but of chance individual actions. But this was a free discussion, in the course of which they did not accuse me but tried to persuade me—a surprising turn of events. I had no idea what sort of people they were or what they were after. In my innocence I presumed it was a kind of a trial and was pleasantly surprised by its free atmosphere, with the accused himself accusing while the judges tried to argue and change his mind. Since their attempts had little effect on me and since I grew particularly excited when speaking about acts of discrimination against Jewish youth, the presiding colonel made another attempt to make me see reason. "Why are you so concerned with Jewish young people? You have a Russian education, your native language is Russian." I realized that this was an attempt to draw me into the camp of the centrists regarding the Jewish question, to convert me to "Christian thinking" and thus eradicate the tenets of "Jewish bourgeois nationalism." But I insisted on my right to protest against the injustice toward Jewish youth, refusing to catch at this straw.

I must say that at the time I had a very vague notion of what Jewish bourgeois nationalism actually was and believed it to be the same as Zionism. It was only later that the implications of the slogan became clear. Soviet Jews had no right openly to be proud of their outstanding compatriots—scientists, composers, artists—for this was a manifestation of Jewish bourgeois nationalism; Jews had no right to be proud of their compatriots' active participation in the revolutionary struggle, for this was a manifestation of Jewish bourgeois nationalism; Jews must not mention their role in fighting Nazism in World War II or be proud of their numerous war heroes, for this was a manifestation of Jewish bourgeois nationalism; it was particularly criminal for Soviet Jews to take pride in the heroism of the resistance fighters in the Warsaw ghetto. Even Anne Frank's *Diary*, published around the world, came out in the Soviet Union later than anywhere else and in such a small edition that it was quickly and permanently sold out. In other words, Jews as an ethnic group were denied the right enjoyed by every national or ethnic minority on earth—the right to take pride in their heroes. Long-standing discrimination has not infrequently instilled an inferiority complex in Jews. So it is sometimes with a certain reluctance that a Jew will say that he is a Jew, as if there were something compromising in such an admission.

I was raised and educated in the Russian culture, in all its aspects: literature, poetry, painting, music, theater. It has always filled my inner life with meaning, and many Jewish intellectuals would say the same. But if all the nationalities and ethnic groups of the Soviet Union take pride in their heroes, why can't the Jews? "I am a Jew by birth, and all my life I have been denigrated for it. Why can't the Jews' contributions to our country's progress be a matter of pride without being branded as Jewish bourgeois nationalism?" I asked my interlocutors.

After we had exhausted the Jewish question, they asked me to characterize Miron Vovsi. I repeated more or less what I had told the general on the night of March 14, only in more detail. I expressed my high opinion of Vovsi as a scientist and therapist and mentioned that we, his friends, had always regretted that he devoted so much time to his medical practice at the expense of his research; but it was not really his fault because he was in great demand as a physician, he was a victim of his tremendous popularity. I told them how staggered I was to learn of his alleged crimes, quite incompatible with his nature, particularly in light of the supposed vigilance of state security organs with respect to a man in the position of chief surgeon to the Soviet Army. I insisted that, despite the fact that he had pleaded guilty, all the accusations against him were absurdities. When I said that I knew of only one debatable flaw in his otherwise spotless life, my audience pricked up their ears. I said that he had tried to buy a cooperative flat for a woman, probably his mistress. Fortunately the affair did not go far, to the great relief of his friends. But my audience was not interested in Vovsi's private life. They waved the matter aside and asked me to concentrate on his political profile—but there was nothing more I could add to that. I realized the naiveté of mentioning Miron Vovsi's intimate affairs in the context of our conference, but I did it on purpose—to emphasize that it was the only compromising detail I knew about the man.

The "trial" made a favorable impression on me, especially since I never expected anything good from the organization that held me captive. I did not feel like an accused man—I was on equal terms with the judges. Only much later, when all the circumstances of the winding up of the doctors' case came to light, did I learn that I was then present not at a trial but at a sitting of the government commission set up to review the plot cooked up by the MGB. This commission was one of the first measures of the new Soviet government to do away with the Stalinist terror; and it was followed by a series of other measures to restore normal life in the country. Perhaps I was already more or less prepared mentally to comment frankly on the negative aspects of our public and academic life. In any case, the atmosphere of this session inspired me to be unreservedly outspoken. By its end I felt I had fully acquitted myself, although no resolution or verdict was pronounced. I had the impression, on the strength of the general spirit of the discussion, that my future would not be so terrible after all. Yet when I asked the colonel outright if I would be returned to normal life as a Soviet citizen, he answered: "This will depend on you, on how you will look at what has happened to you." His answer was unclear to me, leaving scope for all sorts of interpretations. What did he mean? Imprisonment, concentration camp, exile? The idea of liberation had not even crossed my mind; it was quite improbable in Stalin's times. How could I have known that Stalinism had come to an end? During the following days, I tried desperately to figure out what was behind the colonel's words. I would have to summon all my patience and wait to see what would happen.

I had two more brief meetings with the colonel. I think they must have taken place in Lefortovo Prison, where I was returned after the trial. At one of them the colonel asked me to put in written form my testimony that I had always been a loyal Soviet citizen. He did not specify what I was to write about, but merely said: "Well, you know yourself what is expected of you." I understood that they needed material for my rehabilitation, so I wrote about my academic work and research and how much joy I derived from both, and that I had been given this opportunity for fulfillment only thanks to the Soviet system. At our second, brief, meeting, he gave me a list of people and suggested that I renounce the evidence concerning them that I had allegedly given during the investigation. Some of the names on the list had never come up, nor had I ever given libelous evidence against anyone. Still I agreed to do this without arguing, for I understood that it was necessary for their rehabilitation.

So I had to wait. I fretted, but tried to be patient. Again there was a succession of quiet days filled only with reading books from the prison library. My nervous tension did not let up for a second. Particularly unbearable were the nights with persistent insomnia, although now I was allowed to sleep as much as I liked. One day at the end of March or perhaps early April, a pretty young woman doctor entered my cell followed by the guard—the one who was more humane than the others. He tried to persuade me to go to bed each time he saw me sitting up at night. I thought it was he who had brought the doctor (a neuropathologist), but later I understood that she came for quite a different reason. "What's your problem?" she asked me in a somewhat familiar tone. I answered that my main problem was beyond her competence or the circumstances. She ignored the sarcasm and started testing me for elementary neurological reactions. She led me to the window to observe the reaction of my pupils to light and asked me if I had ever had syphilis. I answered her question with another: "Do you note any anisocoria? The pupils react differently to light, don't they?" She answered in the affirmative, and I explained to her that for thirty years I had worked daily with a microscope for many hours, which was the reason for my eye condition. I asked her to prescribe me some Bekhterev tablets for insomnia. She promised to do it, and for the rest of my stay there I received two Bekhterev tablets daily.

After I was released from prison and learned more about the whole affair, I realized that this examination was unlike the one to which I was subjected at the military registration office shortly before my arrest, when they simply wanted to determine the degree of my physical fitness for arrest and imprisonment. Now they probably wanted to establish the degree of my fitness before release from prison, lest my physical condition provide compromising evidence against the establishment in which I had been held. The government statement published soon after these events mentioned coercive measures, "strictly forbidden by law," which had been used to extract evidence from the victims of the Doctors' Plot.

- 9 -

Liberation

AT LONG LAST came the unforgettable day of April 3. It was late afternoon, and I was sitting on the bed reading an interesting book of which subsequent events ousted all memory from my mind. I only remember being so absorbed in it that I tore myself away reluctantly when my prison guard burst into the cell and ordered me quickly to collect my things. He even helped me stuff everything into the pillowcase in which he brought the possessions that had been taken away from me upon my arrival. We put in the remains of the foodstuffs (a piece of smoked sausage, some biscuits, a half loaf of rye bread, several onions) that I had bought with my own money from the prison food vendor. My guard had no idea what lay in store for me, and least of all could he suppose that I would be set free, for that had never before happened to an inmate of Lefortovo Prison. When I asked him if I should take the bread too, he said: "Take everything. You'll need everything there."

Having collected my few prison belongings, we went downstairs where I changed into my own clothes, which now hung loose on me. As it turned out, I had lost 14 kilograms in prison. "I've left my paunch here," I observed, and the guard answered: "Better than a spa treatment, isn't it? So you wanted a good life, eh?" "My life was good enough before I landed here with you." After this exchange of witticisms, I squeezed into the vertical box in a Black Raven and took a seat, my bundle on my knees.

Judging by the preparations, I was leaving my cosy cell for good, or at least I hoped so. In Stalin's day, a person constantly expected all sorts of reversals of fortune. He could never be sure how long his luck would last. As I was leaving my cell, I experienced a complex gamut of feelings, which included all the suffering I went through there, the numerous impressions and observations accumulated during my stay in that house of the dead, and fear of what awaited me on the outside. Strangely enough, there was also an element of sadness: after all I was leaving at that place part of my heart and soul. What I had lived through in that cell was sufficient for a lifetime. And now from imminent violent death, from madness and hell, I hoped I was going toward a return to life.

From the now familiar inner yard of the Lubyanka building, I was taken to the hall and pushed into the box, complete with my bundle. Some time passed (I couldn't say how much, for only my heartbeats marked the minutes), and then I heard a telephone ringing and my name spoken by the officer on duty. The door of the box opened and a captain with a gloomy, pock-marked face called me out for interrogation. The officer on duty was most solicitous and advised me to use the toilet downstairs because the interrogation might last till 5:00 in the morning and I wouldn't be able to use the toilet upstairs. In all probability, only a very limited number of Lubyanka's officers knew the real reason for my presence there. The pock-marked captain took me upstairs in an elevator, and then I entered, alone, a spacious room where I was met by a stocky, graying general who greeted me warmly and offered me his hand. I shook his hand in return thinking that this augured well. There were a desk and two armchairs in the room, a table with a carafe of water and chairs on either side. The general asked me to sit down and, to my query as to which seat I should take, made an expansive gesture with his hand, indicating that I could take any seat, including his own behind his desk. I sat down on one of the chairs at the table with the carafe, after which the general inquired after my health: "How are you feeling, Yakov Lvovich?" I answered him, somewhat heatedly: "How do you think a man in my position should feel?" The general looked at me sympathetically, as it seemed to me, paced the room several times, and at last said: "Well, I had you brought here to inform you that you have been completely exonerated and will be released today."

This news was too much for me, and I broke into tears. All the bitterness of the past months and the shock of this unexpected finale found release in those tears. But I soon managed to control myself. I had a glass of water that the general kindly offered me. To cheer me up, he added: "I have arranged for you to be brought home by car, but first there are some bureaucratic formalities to attend to; they will take about an hour and a half [his tone conveyed the apology, probably feigned, that formalities are inevitable]. Give your family a call from the downstairs telephone to let them know you're coming." I was still unable to believe it was all real and not some game and, to make sure, I probed him: "But what about the alleged Jewish crimes?" The general waved his hand impatiently as if to say that I should forget about them. I asked him how they expected me to behave after what had happened—should I keep quiet about my arrest? The general said: "Your arrest was unlawful and groundless, so you can behave accordingly." After this he said goodbye and wished me well, though I don't remember what he said specifically. The pock-marked captain led me down the long corridors. I was muttering something, and I probably looked dazed with happiness, because the captain's stony face relaxed into the semblance of a smile.

The bureaucratic formalities started with another wait in a box on some upper floor, where I sat in blissful confusion with no inkling as to what was going on. "I'd rip out bureaucracy's guts, I would"—I recalled a line from Mayakovsky, thinking that I myself would not spare my teeth if I had a chance. The time wore on. I could hear the sounds of activity and some voices as I waited eagerly for the door to open. At long last it did, and another officer took me into a room the size of an auditorium, with many desks scattered haphazardly about. They were occupied by young colonels. One of them handed me a certificate, while the others stared with obvious interest as if this were an unusual spectacle. The certificate was typewritten and dated April 3, 1953. I would like to quote it in full, for it was the first in the endless series of similar certificates that followed. But unlike my certificate, which was typewritten, the later certificates were printed forms with a standard text. Here is what it said:

Certificate

Issued to citizen Rapoport, Yakov Lvovich, born 1898, to testify that from February 3, 1953, to April 3, 1953, he was under examination at the former Ministry of State Security of the USSR.

In accordance with Article 4, Paragraph 5, of the Criminal Code of the RSFSR, proceedings instituted against Rapoport, Yakov Lvovich, have been dismissed. He is released from custody and completely rehabilitated.

A. Kuznetsov
Department Chief,
USSR Ministry of the Interior

"The *former* Ministry of State Security"—this phrase hit me in a flash of light. So the MGB had been liquidated? While I was shut up in prison, something momentous must have taken place, which had also effected this dramatic change in my own destiny. I understood that all at once, but what precisely had happened I could not possibly know. After I read the certificate, they returned to me all the documents confiscated during the search of my apartment: my passport, doctoral diploma, certificate for war medals, professorship certificate, and party card. The latter was even more significant as a symbol of liberation than the release certificate itself, for it meant not only rehabilitation in the criminal sense but in the sociopolitical sense as well. It meant that I had been reinstated in the party.

Despite all those papers—the proof of my liberation—I was again sent back to the box. The wheels of the bureaucratic machine were still turning, and although all the preceding events were convincing enough, I was still gripped by that fear which had become so deeply ingrained into all of us during Stalin's reign: what if they change their minds at the last moment? What if some powerful hand turns back the wheel of fortune, and all those papers make a reverse journey and so do I? Twice the door was opened and again locked. The first time they brought the bundle that I had left in the downstairs box; the second time they unlocked the door to inquire if my eyeglass case was in the bundle, for they couldn't find it. I recall having a cheap old cardboard case, which could have been thrown out as a piece of rubbish. Now I was afraid they would keep me there until they found it. So as not to complicate the situation further and to discourage their overconcern for my junk, I told them there was no case. But I marveled at this scrupulous attention to detail—this establishment really had order, to whatever ends it was put.

The long wait was wearing my patience thin; my excitement mounted. I still thought something might reverse my luck. The general had promised that the bureaucratic formalities would take an hour and a half, but I had already been there much longer. So I plucked up my courage and started banging on the door. Soon it opened, and an officer who looked very busy said to me quickly: "Wait a bit more, will you? It won't take long now." I said I might have a heart attack from the stress of waiting, but he only repeated: "Have a bit more patience. It won't take much longer." He was obviously in a hurry to get back to what he had been doing. Even through the closed door, I could sense the hustle and bustle of the busy office full of officers laden with work. Soon I was banging on the door again, this time kicking it in exasperation. The officer who opened the door told me they wanted to return all the valuables confiscated during the search in my flat, so I would not have to come and collect them, and it would take some more time. I had no idea what he was talking about, since I had no valuables at home. But I had to be resigned. A little later the door opened again, and I was led into a room where a service colonel gave me a packet of bonds and the war decorations confiscated at my arrest. These were the valuables that had caused the delay. I immediately picked out my Order of Lenin and fixed it to my lapel. It occurred to me that this would help convince my wife that my liberation was real, before she read the rehabilitation certificate. Thus adorned with the Order of Lenin and carrying my other decorations in my pocket, I was locked in the box again. I don't think this box had ever received an Order-bearing prisoner before: undoubtedly a sign of change.

It was already about two o'clock in the morning when a middle-aged colonel appeared at the door and announced that he was to escort me home. A young plainclothes officer stood behind him. When I tried to pick up my bundle, the colonel ordered the young man to get it for me, and he hurried to obey. The three of us moved in a file led by the colonel with some paper in his hand on which I caught sight of my prison photograph: the front view and the profile. I followed the colonel, and the procession was brought up by the young man carrying my bundle. On each floor, the officer on duty checked the paper, which must have been a no-return pass. They did not allow me to call home from the downstairs telephone. In the courtyard, a large gray car was waiting. The colonel and I sat in the back, while the young man with the bundle took the front seat. The gates of Lubyanka opened, and I started on my journey home.

It is difficult to describe what I felt during that ride across nocturnal Moscow, which for decades had been wreathed in blood-curdling legends, as I made my way back from the netherworld, a world full of horrible mysteries. It may seem that escape from it would be sure to cause an emotional explosion, but there was none. I only felt serene delight in the deserted but well-lit Moscow streets, in the familiar buildings, the neon advertisements in Gorky Street. It was like meeting old friends. I felt happy to see them all in place and anticipated each memorable sight: the Moscow City Soviet, the Yeliseyev supermarket, the monument to Pushkin . . . They symbolized, as it were, the permanence of everyday life, quite alien to the phantasmagoria in which I had been immersed. I was blissfully conscious of the fact that I was going—not being transported—home, that I could stop the car and get out. I felt like a person waking up from a horrible nightmare into the real, familiar world. I no longer doubted that I was, indeed, on my way home: down Gorky Street and Leningrad Avenue we approached Novopeshchanaya Street where I lived. I was even glad that the car was moving slowly, as if the driver had guessed my wish. I had always enjoyed Moscow at night with its quiet streets and scarce pedestrians. And now this encounter with Moscow right after Lefortovo and Lubyanka seemed like a fairy tale. In prison, I often recited the meaningful concluding verses from Blok's "Retribution." They again came to mind on my way home, and I would like to quote them here:

> When through the city's wilderness,
> Eyelashes caked with icy rime,
> In body and in mind depressed,
> You slowly make your way back home . . .
> Just pause, no matter where you are,
> Listen to night's tranquillity;
> Sounds of life come to your ear
> That you have never heard by day . . .
> And you will bless all things that are,
> Knowing that life itself means more,
> Much more than Brand's "All or nothing,"
> And that this world is ever fair.

The psychological ease with which I switched over to the living world after the nightmare of Lubyanka and Lefortovo was amazing. Their horrors were melting away as the real world entered my consciousness. My memory held on to most of the events of the past months, but they were pushed into my subconscious by the powerful new impressions. Life would probably be impossible if the human mind did not possess this miraculous capacity for adaptation and survival. No human being is capable of bearing a heavy load of negative emotions for long.

Alas, I could not be alone with my thoughts in the car. My two companions were a sign of special attention toward an innocently maligned professor. One of them, the middle-aged colonel who sat next to me, kept complaining of a pain in his heart, for which I gave him medical advice. He reminded me of the other colonel who took me away to Lubyanka on that night of February 3. The other companion, who sat in the front seat with my bundle, seemed familiar to me. I suspected I had seen this hostile face with the forced smile on the MGB agent who met me and my wife on the night of the arrest and searched my pockets so dexterously. I asked him about it, and he confirmed my guess. Then I asked if he had done my wife any harm, and he denied it emphatically. Yet Sophia told me later that he had been the most vicious of the group—so much so that the others had tried to restrain his ardor. That was why he was so sulky. What an anticlimax!

The car turned onto Novopeshchanaya Street, passed through the iron gates into the courtyard, and stopped at my entrance. The three of us got out of the car. It was 3:00 a.m. when we entered the hall, where there was a telephone. The elevators did not work at night. My dog, a black poodle named Topsy, was the first to sense my presence while I was still on the ground floor. She was a remarkably intelligent and emotional dog. Each time I came home, she greeted me with rapturous delight, smothered me with affection accompanied by happy squealing, groaning, and a leak on the floor. Before I had time to telephone my wife and warn her of my arrival, lest the sight of the two MGB men frighten her, she was awakened by Topsy's barking: my dog was the first to announce to the world the end of the Doctors' Plot. We went up to the third floor slowly, out of consideration for the colonel's bad heart. I unbuttoned my coat so that my wife could see the Order of Lenin at once, as a sign of my rehabilitation, and she did notice it the moment she opened the door. But I could only embrace her after Topsy was done with affectionate jumping and I had stepped over the traditional puddle she made on the floor. My companions came in too, but the lieutenant disappeared almost at once. I can't remember what it was my wife and I said to each other in the colonel's presence. During his long career, it was the first time that he had ever taken anyone home from Lubyanka, so no wonder he felt out of his element. He asked permission to make a telephone call, and I heard him reporting to the general: "Comrade General, I'm calling from Yakov Lvovich's apartment." In response to the general's question, he said: "Both joy and tears." Then he conveyed the general's regards and the wish that from now on we would have only joys without tears. It was all very moving.

My wife asked me if I knew that Stalin had died. This immediately put everything into place in the hitherto incomprehensible series of events. Now I understood why the MGB was called "former" in my rehabilitation certificate. It occurred to me that Fate had chosen that particular moment to strike him down so that my life might be spared. But why had she waited so long? Why had she allowed so many millions of other lives to be lost? My wife asked me cautiously if I knew anything about Miron Vovsi. I said that all were being set free, since I was sure that a general process of rehabilitation had started with me. (As I had sat locked in the box waiting to be released and listening to the bustle outside, I thought I heard Vovsi's name being pronounced in a whisper. At the time I visualized him being led down the corridor and somebody pointing him out as the main culprit in the Doctors' Plot—a villain who deserved to be hung, drawn, and quartered.) The colonel's presence was a nuisance, although he tried to keep in the background and was himself embarrassed at being one too many at my reunion with my wife. He had to wait for the lieutenant, who had gone down to fetch the house manager to remove the seals from the two rooms in his presence and reinstate me as the owner of my rooms with all their contents. The two must have received instructions to carry out all the formalities on the spot. This was thoughtful of them, because the MGB was never in a hurry to unseal rooms in such cases, which were far and few between in any case. In this instance, they obviously wanted to remove all traces of the arrest.

The house manager later told me that when he was awakened that night by the lieutenant, whom he remembered well in connection with my arrest, he had no doubts that they had come to arrest my wife. In his agitation, he could not get his legs into his trousers, but when the lieutenant informed him in a cheerless tone that they had brought me back, he cried out: "Let's run then!" And they ran to my apartment, removed all the seals and I entered my rooms, which were in a state of utter chaos from the search. Having completed all the formalities connected with reinstating me and restoring my rights, the colonel cordially took his leave, wishing all the best to me and my wife.

At long last, I was left alone with Sophia, and I really felt I was home. I could walk from one room to another, go into the bathroom or kitchen without asking permission, just as the fancy struck me. It was only then that I became fully aware of the freedom I had regained. My wife tried to persuade me to go to bed, but I wanted to prolong the exhilarating feeling of freedom, my enjoyment over the return to normal life and familiar objects. I was so excited I wouldn't be able to sleep anyway; it would have seemed a violation of my freedom. I went to the bathroom for a shave. Not that I needed it, but I wanted to experience the sheer joy of using my own razor, my own mirror, my own towel. These objects were also symbols of freedom. Then I sent an express cable by telephone to my elder daughter in Toropets. Such cables are supposed to reach the addressee in one hour, but mine arrived twelve hours later. I informed her in the cable that I had "returned from my business trip," but my daughter called me before she received the cable, immediately after she heard on the radio that the doctors' case had been closed. The local authorities were probably quite confused: only yesterday these doctors had been villains and enemies of the people. So they had decided to wait for further information before delivering my cable.

Then came the memorable morning of April 4. At 6:00 a.m., instead of the morning news, the full text of the official government announcement about the end of the Doctors' Plot was broadcast. It deserves to be quoted in full:

Announcement
of the USSR Ministry of the Interior
April 4, 1953

The USSR Ministry of the Interior has carefully examined all materials of the investigation and related data concerning a group of doctors accused of sabotage, espionage, and other subversive activities aimed at doing harm to certain Soviet leaders. It has been established that the arrests of the doctors allegedly involved in this plot—Professor M. S. Vovsi, Professor V. N. Vinogradov, Professor M. B. Kogan, Professor B. B. Kogan, Professor P. I. Yegorov, Professor A. I. Feldman, Professor Ya. G. Etinger, Professor V. Kh. Vasilenko, Professor A. M. Grinstein, Professor V. F. Zelenin, Professor B. S. Preobrazhensky, Professor N. A. Popova, Professor V. V. Zakusov, Professor N. A. Shershevsky, and Dr. G. I. Mayorov—by the former Ministry of State Security, were illegal and completely unjustified.

It has been established that the accusations against the above persons are false and the documentary materials non-authentic. All evidence given by the accused, who allegedly pleaded guilty, was forced from them by the investigators of the former Ministry of State Security with methods strictly forbidden by Soviet law.

On the basis of the considered decision of the special commission set up by the Ministry of the Interior to check the circumstances of the case, the arrested persons—M. S. Vovsi, V. N. Vinogradov, B. B. Kogan, P. I. Yegorov, A. I. Feldman, V. Kh. Vasilenko, A. M. Grinstein, V. F. Zelenin, B. S. Preobrazhensky, N. A. Popova, V. V. Zakusov, N. A. Shershevsky, G. I. Mayorov, and others involved in this case—have been completely exonerated as regards the accusations of sabotage, espionage, and terrorism, and released from custody in accordance with Article 4, Paragraph 5, of the Criminal Code of the RSFSR.

The persons guilty of mishandling the investigation have been arrested, and criminal proceedings have been instituted against them.

This historical document was printed in the official newspapers alongside other articles with headings typical of those days: "Spring in Michurin Orchards," "Travels Around Our Native Land," and "Workers Raise Their Cultural Level." At the bottom of the same page was the following announcement: "The Presidium of the USSR Supreme Soviet has resolved to abolish the decree of January 20, 1953, awarding Dr. Lydia Timashuk the Order of Lenin. The award has been declared invalid in connection with fresh evidence that has since come to light." In this way, Timashuk was demoted from being a "great daughter of the Russian people" to a run-of-the-mill MGB agent.

The arrangement of these two announcements on the newspaper page—one at the top and the other at the bottom—was not accidental, for it was the same both in *Pravda* and *Izvestiya*, the two major dailies, the only difference being in the dividing articles and their headings. The aim of such an arrangement was to tone down the sensational nature of both announcements, to make them look quite ordinary, nothing more than regular measures being taken by the new government. This becomes particularly evident if we compare the text of the decree awarding Timashuk the Order of Lenin—printed on the front page in large type—with the modest note about the annullment of the award done in small type. Still, these ruses could not conceal the importance of the two announcements, which were without precedent in the history of the Soviet state, particularly the statement about the exoneration of persons accused of heinous crimes, who had pleaded guilty in the course of the MGB investigation but who were cleared nevertheless. Not only were a large number of innocent people snatched from the jaws of ignoble death and their good names restored, but also that announcement was virtually a condemnation of the entire thirty-six years of Stalin's tyranny. It spotlighted the worst aspects of Stalin's regime: its monstrous arbitrary rule and the mechanism of fabricating various plots allegedly disclosed thanks to the vigilance of the security bodies. Untold numbers of people, including the finest representatives of the Communist Party and the Soviet people, were declared enemies of the people, and even greater numbers—their families and relatives—were reduced to lives of misery and privation. That historical decision passed a verdict on Stalin's regime and marked the start of an all-round restructuring of Soviet society.

Of great interest is *Pravda*'s commentary on the Ministry of the Interior's announcement of April 4, 1953, which was printed on April 6 and reprinted in full on April 7 by *Izvestiya* and other newspapers under the headline: "Soviet Socialist Law Is Inviolable." The text of the original announcement about the release of the doctors was followed by the question: "How was it possible that the Ministry of State Security, bound to protect the interests of the Soviet state, was responsible for a framed-up case victimizing honest Soviet citizens and outstanding scientists?" The article gave an exhaustive answer to the question, which I paraphrase closely:

1. MGB leaders failed in their duty; they alienated themselves from the people and forgot that they were supposed to serve them.

2. Former MGB Minister Ignatyev was guilty of political

blindness and negligence. He let himself be misinformed by such criminal adventurists as former Deputy Minister Ryumin, who personally supervised the investigation. Ryumin, now under arrest, acted as a covert enemy of the people and the state. Instead of denouncing real spies and saboteurs, he chose the path of falsehood and adventurism; thus he violated the law and the constitution.

3. The medical commission set up in connection with the Doctors' Plot failed in their duty as well and made erroneous conclusions regarding the treatment of Shcherbakov and Zhdanov. Instead of examining the case histories and other relevant materials with scientific conscientiousness and objectiveness, the commission allowed itself to be misled by faked evidence and thus supported with its professional authority the slanderous and false accusations against noted medical scientists. (The article tried to smooth over somewhat the reproof addressed to the examination commission by mentioning that certain important details of the medical treatment were concealed from them, details that proved its correctness.)

The editorial further censured despicable adventurists of the Ryumin type who attempted to fan national enmity (antisemitism), which was completely alien to Soviet society. They did not stop at slander. Thus they had defamed Mikhoels, the outstanding stage director and a prominent public figure. In conclusion, the article urged strict observation of the law and the constitution.

The courage and civic awareness exhibited by the new government so soon after it replaced Stalin's regime must be admired—all the more so because the social climate at the time of the Doctors' Plot and public opinion throughout the country would have led to a completely different outcome. It was necessary to enlighten the public as to the circumstances of the case and reveal the culprits responsible for its fabrication. To put it all down to the ill will of the adventurist Ryumin, the blind gullibility of Minister Ignatyev, and the inefficiency of the medical examination commission might seem superficial. But some sort of explanation was urgently needed before a deeper analysis could be made of the historical circumstances that permitted Stalin's tyranny. An open admission of the arbitrary and lawless nature of the Stalinist regime was made at the Twentieth Party Congress and reaffirmed by the release of huge numbers of political prisoners and mass rehabilitations, mostly posthumous.

The criticism of the role of the medical examination commission contained in the *Pravda* and *Izvestiya* editorials is of special relevance to the Doctors' Plot. One can only feel disgust at the servile readiness of the commission to flout medical ethics, dating back to the time of Hippocrates, and to sacrifice dozens of their finest colleagues in order to get into the MGB's good books. These professors turned out to be no better than Ryumin and his kind. The latter were professional agents whose careers depended on the number of victims exterminated, while the former were supposed to represent the most humane of professions. Their complicity is further evidence of the general moral decay in Soviet society of the time. Even the medical profession could not avoid the corrupting effects of Stalin's regime. That the members of the commission quickly renounced their own conclusions after the new government had established their falseness arouses even stronger disgust, for it indicates a complete lack of professional integrity.

The withdrawal of a government award from a person recently decorated, and the announcement of the fact in the press with an explanation of the reasons for the annulment, was also without precedent, and it gave rise to all sorts of rumors about the fate of the person thus treated: Lydia Timashuk. The most widespread was that she had met with a fatal car accident, a story that is still favored by some. It seemed quite plausible at the time, especially considering the sinister rumors that the MGB often did away with people in this fashion, Mikhoels for one. Nothing of the sort happened to Timashuk. Shortly after the April events, she resumed work at the Kremlin Hospital where she had wrought such havoc. She reappeared in her office, apparently unperturbed, as if none of this had had anything to do with her—as if nothing, in fact, had happened. Perhaps she had been advised to behave in this way. Shortly afterwards, when a group of doctors was nominated for government awards, she was included in the list to be awarded the Order of the Red Banner of Labor, second in importance to the Order of Lenin. Apparently her reputation was not considered besmirched by her abortive attempt to pose as Joan of Arc. Her actions were probably classified as vigilance and patriotic zeal, which had always been encouraged (and still are). And if her zeal misfired—who is without sin among us?

But let us go back to my apartment on the morning of April 4. After the radio announcement, neighbors flocked to our apartment despite the early hour. The first to come was Nina Beklemisheva (whom I have already mentioned) and her husband Vladimir. They had been unable to sleep all night, listening to the noises from our apartment and the sound of many feet. They knew that only my wife and younger daughter were supposed to be in the apartment and were convinced that the MGB had come to arrest them too. They were overjoyed by the radio announcement, so Nina rushed to break the good news to my wife. When she saw me, she burst into uncontrollable sobbing, an effect of all the mental anguish caused her by the Doctors' Plot and my arrest. The news of my return quickly spread about the building. Through the window I saw people crowding around the house manager, who was telling everyone about my arrival. Our doorbell kept ringing, and I heard my wife telling people that I was too tired to see anyone. But our neighbors insisted on taking just one look at me and she couldn't refuse them. In their eyes I was a symbol of liberation. And certainly I was happy to see them as well. Many could not hold back their tears. These people, both Russians and Jews, had themselves lived in constant fear of arrest. Now they wanted to see with their own eyes the proof of what had been announced over the radio.

In the morning, before working hours, I called up the Tarasevich Institute's director, Semyon Didenko, to inform him of my release, but he already knew about it. He begged me to come to the institute for at least half an hour, so people could see me there in person. But he asked me to wait until after noon, and later I understood why: in my absence, my laboratory had been closed down and its premises were occupied by another department. So Didenko, a sensitive man, wanted time to put everything in order, the way it had been before my arrest—especially my own small office. And indeed I found all my subordinates in their former places and my office in its usual state—only the floor was still wet from the recent scrubbing. On my desk I found a circular reinstating me to my former position as head of the laboratory of pathologic morphology, with back pay due for the entire period of my absence.

When I came to the institute that morning, I was taken aback by the cool and matter-of-course manner of the people I met in the halls—even those who used to greet me enthusiastically. Didenko explained the reason for this: earlier that morning, the institute's party secretary, Anna Tebyakina, had been summoned to the District Party Committee, where they informed her of my release and asked her to instruct party members, and through them the other employees, to receive me as if I had returned from a business trip, with no emotional outbursts. The instruction was strictly observed, in marked contrast to the exaggerated attention I was accorded during the release procedures at Lubyanka. The instruction reflected the district committee's confusion in the face of the unexpected developments. They did not know how they were supposed to react and decided to follow the French rule: "When in doubt, do nothing." How could the district committee and the institute party members be expected suddenly to change their attitudes when only a short time ago they had been branding me as a murdering villain? The overnight change had taken them unawares.

When I had informed Didenko by telephone about my intention to come to the institute, he asked me to wait in my office till he summoned me, for he wanted to see me alone, without witnesses. Free then to ignore the district committee's instructions, he greeted me with embraces and tears. He also told me that only the day before, on Friday, there had been a party bureau meeting at which he had been accused of supporting an enemy of the people for a number of years. The discussion dragged on into the night and was adjourned until Monday, when a resolution was to be taken (probably the resolution had already been drawn up and would hardly have been favorable for Didenko). But the next day, on Saturday, the enemy of the people appeared at the institute with a certificate of complete rehabilitation. That was no doubt quite enough to shock the institute's party leadership. A similar shock was experienced by many trigger-happy zealots who thrived under Stalin's relentless rule. My daughter in Toropets told me later how, that morning, the enraged party secretary of the out-patient clinic where she worked burst into her office shouting: "Have you heard? They've been released! This is a foul provocation! They will answer for it!" Obviously, the preparations for winding up the doctors' case had been carried out in complete secrecy, strictly within the confines of the Ministry of the Interior. The guard at Lefortovo, who saw me out of the prison, did not know where I was going. Moreover, even the officer on duty at Lubyanka did not know why I had been brought there. Otherwise, why would he have advised me to use the downstairs toilet before what he thought was going to be a long interrogation?

There had been some signs of the coming change, I later found out, and one such was a telephone call to my wife several days before my release. A man's voice greeted her politely and inquired after her health. He introduced himself as an MGB officer and inquired after the health of the other members of my family, allegedly on my behalf. My wife said to reassure me that all was well and that she had obtained work, doing translations and abstracts of articles from scientific journals (my wife is a physiologist). When she asked how I was, she was told that

"Yakov Lvovich is quite well." My wife asked if she could send me a lighter coat, for it was spring and I had left in my winter coat. But the man replied that there was no need. My wife failed to grasp the hidden message contained in this remark, to see it as a signal of my impending return. The Soviet reality of those days gave little reason for optimism. Rather, having heard that similar telephone calls had been made as a reward to the prisoner for cooperating with the investigation, my wife decided that the call had been made in my presence as a reward for admitting guilt. It appears that, just as the neuropathologist examined me to establish my fitness for returning home, they also wanted to establish the fitness of my family for receiving me.

During my first day at the institute, I had a call from the doorman downstairs who informed me that an officer wanted to see me. This did not shake me in the least—such was the great psychological change I had undergone in only a few hours. I asked the doorman to conduct the man to my office. He turned out to be a MGB colonel, bringing back the materials confiscated during the search of my office after my arrest. He found me peering into the microscope and was evidently impressed by my quick transformation from a prisoner into a scientist at work. I heard him reporting by telephone to the general that he had returned my materials and that he had found me engrossed in my work. His voice conveyed a mixture of amazement and admiration. I was glad that, thanks to Didenko, I was able to demonstrate to the MGB bosses that they could not kill devotion to science with their handcuffs. Nor was I showing off. My strongest desire while in prison had been to get back to that microscope, and so almost the first thing I did upon taking possession of my office was to study a couple of interesting histological preparations made during my absence. I was not the only erstwhile prisoner who couldn't wait to get back to work. Miron Vovsi, despite a general indisposition after his ordeals, could not be persuaded to rest even one day before resuming his lectures at the Refresher Medical Institute.

The colonel was not the last MGB officer I had to deal with. Soon after I came back from the institute, there was a telephone call from Lubyanka to find out if I was at home and if I could receive a messenger from them. I was tickled pink—imagine their asking my permission before sending an officer over. Only two months before, they had come without asking and learned about my whereabouts from their own agents. I gave my permission, though I had no idea of the purpose of the visit. A young lieutenant, good-looking and well-mannered, brought papers that had been confiscated during the search of my apartment. There was a sackful of them, and I suggested that he dump them right on the floor in my study so I could sort them out later. A little mound of paper formed, but I had no time to sort anything out just then. I simply stuffed the papers into my bookcase and desk drawers. Most of those papers remained untouched until many years later, when I found many interesting and long-forgotten documents. I exchanged a few amiable remarks with the lieutenant, who showed a young person's respect toward a professor and scientist. I mentioned in passing that my investigator now probably regretted that he had not believed my protestations of innocence. The lieutenant's answer was quite unexpected and full of hidden meaning: if the investigator had believed me then, he said, he wouldn't be in the position he was in now. He asked me if I would like to see him. I refused emphatically; I was not in the least curious about my former investigator. But I understood from the lieutenant's tone that my investigator's position was far from enviable, to the extent that probably we had changed places or, at any rate, he was in some state of distress.

The rest of my first day at home was filled with all sorts of mundane matters connected with the return to normal life. One of them was calling for a doctor from the out-patient polyclinic for scientific personnel from which my family and I had been expelled after my arrest. The doctor came at once and diagnosed very high blood pressure and general emaciation, although the loss of 14 kilograms still left me enough flesh to live on. He advised bed rest, but I was impatient to plunge into my work, so this advice remained one of the many unfulfilled doctors' orders.

On the evening of that first day, our apartment was invaded by friends who came to share our joy and celebrate my release. I greeted them with a line from Pushkin's "Letter to a Friend": "Haggard, close-cropped, but alive I've escaped from Aesculapius." Most of our friends brought some food to add to the modest fare we could offer them. The latter included what I had carried back from the prison: smoked sausage, rye bread, onions, and biscuits. I recalled the prison guard's advice: "Take everything. You'll need everything there." Indeed it all came in handy—only not where he thought it would. Oddly enough, our small feast almost coincided with Easter matins. My return was a veritable resurrection from the dead following a kind of crucifixion. There was much food for philosophical reflection. That blissful first day of freedom!

The elation of that first day gradually gave way to more sobering reactions. Legally, the Doctors' Plot was ended, but it was far from over in the broader political sense. I was aware of its repercussions in both my public and my personal life for quite some time afterwards. Historians and sociologists have yet to make a thorough study of all its aspects, and it has not been treated in any detail in fiction or nonfiction. I will report here only my personal views and the facts at my disposal.

I was flooded with information about events that had occurred during my imprisonment. Jewish doctors, even those who were not arrested, were fiercely attacked, particularly in the pages of *Meditsinsky rabotnik*, which stooped to all sorts of slander, however improbable. Finding herself in financial straits, my wife was forced to sell a few things, and immediately someone informed the MGB that she was selling goods that were to be confiscated after I was sentenced. The MGB men who came to check found that she had been selling only her own possessions, but nonetheless they advised her to stop so as not to provoke the informers.

Since my blood pressure remained at a critical level those first days after my release, I stayed home on sick leave. Apart from the results of my prison experiences, my condition was exacerbated by many irritating events that followed. A few days after my release, I got a call from the secretary of the institute's party organization, who invited me to attend a party meeting to restore my membership. I explained that my membership had already been restored, and my card had been returned, so they needn't bother. But the secretary objected that since the institute's organization had expelled me, according to the rules they had to readmit me. I had never been conversant in the finer aspects of the party rules, but I knew that so-called personal cases, particularly expulsions from the party, could not be considered in the absence of the accused. Under the pretext of illness, I refused to attend the meeting and said that, since they had seen fit to expel me in my absence, they could now restore my membership in my absence. But apparently the ritual had to be observed to the letter, and my presence at that special meeting was imperative. I decided to comply.

The atmosphere at the meeting was unaccountably hostile. It was as if I had robbed these individuals or offended them in some way. The expressions on their faces were more befitting a funeral than a resurrection of an innocent fellow party member. The party secretary repeated to me (privately) some of my alleged utterances, implying that only Stalin's death had saved me and my comrades from the firing squad. When I admitted authorship, she was shattered by my seditious mood and lack of caution, so strong was the Stalinist spirit in those people. Of course they could hardly in a day cleanse their souls of something so deeply ingrained. The party secretary announced the purpose of the meeting: to restore my party membership in light of my complete rehabilitation and reinstatement at my job. All those present obediently voted for the proposal, and then it was over.

After a few days of rest, I went to see Alexei Abrikosov. He told me how he had spent the period of the Doctors' Plot. His story deserves special mention, particularly because he was no rank-and-file professor but a scientist of world renown, a member of the Academy of Sciences and the Academy of Medical Sciences, bearer of the Stalin Prize and the title of Hero of Socialist Labor. For him the doctors' business began long before it assumed its full scope. Suffice it to say that he had a Jewish wife, Fanny Wulf, a pathologist at the Kremlin Hospital where Abrikosov was a consultant. They were both released from duty at the hospital as soon as arrests among the senior medical personnel began. Many others were discharged as well. At first Abrikosov had no idea why. It was not the custom in those days to give reasons, and the dismissed people were lost in conjectures about what they might have done wrong or how they had displeased their superiors. There is always something sinister about an unmotivated dismissal.

Further developments bred anxiety even in Abrikosov, ordinarily a calm and philosophical man. He related his story in his usual composed manner. The Abrikosovs lived on Novoslobodskaya Street, in a building largely inhabited by medical professors, who kept disappearing one after another, transported to less comfortable lodgings—to prison cells. The atmosphere in the building was not at all congenial to friendly contacts, since all the residents were potential candidates for deportation. Moreover, having worked at the Kremlin Hospital, Abrikosov and his wife were considered politically besmirched and were treated with suspicion. So they found themselves in virtual isolation. Even among his colleagues at the department he had headed for more than thirty years, he felt like a pariah. His subordinates stopped coming to him for advice. His office, which used to be visited by all sorts of people, was now deserted, and he spent his working hours in depressing solitude. The department was practically being run by his assistant, Strukov, who was very anxious to uphold his own authority. Any contact with Abrikosov was regarded as a political misdemeanor. Strukov was a man with finely tuned political receptors and was obviously guided in his behavior by considerations of expediency, or maybe he had received direct instructions.

One not so fine day, Abrikosov came to work as usual and found a message on his desk from Talyzin, the institute's rector, summoning him to his office at 3:00. Abrikosov suspected the reason for the summons and had his resignation ready, just in case. Talyzin had also invited the institute's party secretary to the interview. He asked Abrikosov: "I remember you were thinking of resigning your chair. Do you still have such an intention?" This question had only a remote bearing on the actual situation. Several years before, there had been talk that the position of Honorary Professor was to be introduced. A person so titled would be relieved of managing the affairs of the department but would continue his research activities, while receiving the same salary, after the practice of some western universities. Rumor had it that the first professors to receive this title would be Abrikosov and Vinogradov. Abrikosov said openly at the time that he would be happy to accept such an offer if it came: it would have been a reward to an outstanding scientist for many years of fruitful research. But the question asked by Talyzin had very different implications. Abrikosov understood the polite suggestion that he resign, so he produced his application from his briefcase, saying that his intention had not changed.

Of course Abrikosov's plans to resign differed vastly from the way in which it actually occurred: this was no honorable resignation with financial benefits—he was simply being pensioned off. But he had to put a good face on a very bad job. Having obtained Abrikosov's resignation so easily, the rector and the party secretary could not conceal their satisfaction at this unexpectedly simple conclusion to an unpleasant matter. Abrikosov reminded the rector that his dismissal was supposed to be approved by the Committee for Higher Education (later the Ministry of Higher and Secondary Education), which alone could appoint and dismiss professors. The rector and the secretary hastened to assure him that they would see to all the formalities, and he was not to worry. Indeed, they did everything with record speed: half an hour later, when Abrikosov returned to his office, he found on his desk the rector's typewritten order to dismiss him from his post as department head, according to his own wish. Abrikosov never returned to the institute again, and his chair was given to Strukov. This took place at the end of January or early February 1953.

The news of Abrikosov's dismissal from the First Medical Institute quickly spread among the professors and lecturers, along with false rumors of his arrest. At the next sitting of the Academic Council, one of its members, Julia Dombrovskaya, announced the unexpected resignation of Alexei Abrikosov, a veteran professor at the institute, but suggested that he remain on the council. The suggestion was accepted, for it appeared innocent enough and there were no apparent motives for refusal, since Abrikosov had never been openly prosecuted. Having learned that he was still on the council, Abrikosov dutifully attended the next session, where someone's thesis was being considered. After the defense procedure was over, the secretary went around to the council members, handing out voting cards. When she came to Abrikosov, she consulted her list and, not finding him there, bypassed him. Abrikosov understood the implication: Dombrovskaya's suggestion was nothing more than a gesture. So he never attended the council's sittings again, and he was not invited to any.

Abrikosov was then dismissed from the journal *Arkhiv patologii*, which he had founded and had been editing ever since. Soon after he was forced to retire from the institute, he received a telephone message summoning him to see Belousov, deputy minister of health in charge of personnel, who addressed him thus: "Alexei Ivanovich, I understand you've been complaining about your health [Abrikosov had once mentioned his trifacial neuralgia]. Editing *Arkhiv patologii* must be a terrible burden on you." Abrikosov took the hint and said that it was. (He saw no point in contradicting the boss, he explained to me.) Then the deputy minister informed him that the decision had been taken to relieve him of his duties as editor-in-chief and appoint the same Strukov, formerly executive secretary of the journal. Thus Abrikosov was removed from the last of his public and academic posts. It so happened that Strukov fell ill just then, so the journal remained without leadership. The head of the editorial office continued to ask Abrikosov for help, expecting him to solve all the problems, including purely technical ones, which Abrikosov did in the interests of the journal.

Once, quite by chance, Abrikosov met Nikolai Anichkov, president of the Academy of Medical Sciences, in the elevator of the apartment house where they both lived. Anichkov expressed his indignation at Abrikosov's dismissal from his post as editor-in-chief. He said the journal would never be the same without Abrikosov and that he was going to report it to Belousov at the Ministry of Health. Belousov explained to Anichkov that it was beyond his competence to decide such matters and that he would have to consult with the Central Committee of the party. Later he asked Anichkov to pass on to Abrikosov that he was allowed to take care of the journal's affairs temporarily until Strukov recovered.

"You've been treated like a Jew," I commented when I heard Abrikosov's story, intending it as a joke. But Abrikosov agreed with me in all seriousness: "Yes, yes, just like a Jew." God knows what would have happened to Abrikosov if the Doctors' Plot had not ended when it did. All these misadventures were probably a prelude to arrest. Abrikosov's story is typical of stage-by-stage repressions, which, in his case, did not culminate as expected for reasons quite beyond the control of their diabolical inventors. Without a doubt, a case was being concocted against Abrikosov to involve him in the Doctors' Plot. Why was the sword of Damocles suspended above Abrikosov's head? What crime could be imputed to him? According to the MGB's "iron logic," Abrikosov's guilt was obvious since he personally had performed autopsies on leading Soviet statesmen. One was Menzhinsky, chairman of OGPU, in whose body he found no trace of Kazakov's "potion" despite the insistence of the OGPU officer present at the autopsy. He found only advanced sclerosis of coronary arteries, which had caused death. Yet it was announced officially in the statement on the Doctors' Plot that Menzhinsky had been "brutally murdered" by his attending doctors on orders from enemies of the people. Abrikosov also knew the real cause of Ordzhonikidze's death (suicide). The MGB felt it could not rely on his discretion and would rather have this secret sealed safely in the grave along with Abrikosov himself. All of this made Abrikosov a sitting duck. However, in view of his high position and reputation, the MGB needed to prepare public opinion for his downfall. This reminds me for some reason of a Georgian story about a barber who, when he couldn't find his brush, spat on his palm, soaped it, and started spreading the suds on his client's face. In reply to the indignant client's protest, the barber said: "You mustn't be offended. I'm showing you great respect. Usually I spit right into the face of somebody else." Abrikosov was treated with the same sort of respect by the MGB.

I should add here that not all the doctors who had been arrested regained status quo ante on April 4, 1953. The MGB was notorious for its paradoxes. One such involved Mark Sereisky, a noted psychiatrist. He was arrested later than the other doctors, in early March, on the eve of the turning of the tide in the doctors' case. His investigator, as he told me later, wanted him to admit his criminal ties with Vladimir Zelenin, a close friend who figured prominently in the Doctors' Plot. He persisted in his pressure on Sereisky long after Zelenin had been released and was completely rehabilitated. Zelenin was in fact vacationing at a health resort, completely unaware that he was still considered a killer doctor by someone at the MGB and that the hapless Sereisky was being browbeaten to give evidence to that effect. The investigator used such foul language in referring to Zelenin that Sereisky had no doubt the former had already been killed or was about to face the firing squad.

The finale of this macabre story was quite bizarre for Sereisky. At the end of April, instead of the usual interrogation, his investigator asked him just one question: "So you deny that you're shit? Then get the hell out of here!" He was issued an exit pass and released from Lubyanka Prison then and there. He had the feeling he was being thrown out of class for bad behavior rather than being released from prison. So he took a bus home, still in the dark as to the meaning of the farce he had been involved in. As I mentioned earlier, such baffling scenarios were popular among MGB officers, who entertained themselves and polished their creative style at the same time. So far only a small fraction of the information concerning such pointless and often lethal entertainments has been made public, through stories by the few surviving victims and trial materials made accessible in various archives. But massive volumes of it remain unknown.

On April 20, after two weeks of getting back to "normal," my wife and I went on vacation to a sanatorium in Sochi on the Black Sea. The Gelsteins—fellow sufferers in the plot—went there too. Despite the dramatic changes that had occurred in the country and in our personal lives, we still experienced the fear of persecution that we had lived with for decades. We read hidden meaning into random facts and events. For instance, just as we were boarding the train, we heard some cameras clicking and immediately thought we were being photographed by security agents. Naturally we were not alone at the station, so it might have had nothing to do with us, but the habit of being constantly under surveillance was still much too strong for us to ignore such incidents.

On the train another incident occurred that at first alarmed us greatly. On the second day of our journey, the conductor entered our compartment and asked me with some caution (later she explained she did not want to appear intrusive) if my name was Rapoport. My first thought was: "How does she know who I am? Somebody must have informed her, and I can just imagine who that somebody might be." I said that yes, my name was Rapoport and what did she want? She explained that another passenger in our car claimed to have been a student of mine, asked her to see if I was indeed Rapoport and, if I was, to inquire whether he could drop in to see me. I was relieved and asked the conductor to extend a heartfelt welcome to the traveler. Soon he appeared in person, and he turned out to be a specialist in forensic medicine, a celebrity in his field who had indeed been a student of mine and also knew me from my publications in related fields of pathology. We greeted each other warmly, and I accepted his offer to celebrate the meeting with a bottle of cognac, despite my wife's weak protests (I was still suffering from the aftereffects of my imprisonment, particularly hypertension). Other travelers joined our celebration, and the rest of the journey we spent cheering the inner man. But for a long time the cats scalded by Stalin feared even cold water.

That month in Sochi was marked by a spring of rejuvenation both in nature and in my personal life. The first day in the sanatorium, as is often the case, was not a very happy one. We were given an extremely uncomfortable room with windows facing a service yard, with cars and trucks constantly coming in and out, with kitchen smells, a noisy staff, and a public address system to boot. So I slept badly the first night, and my wife quietly went to see the head doctor and asked to be moved to quieter surroundings, considering where I had come from and the nervous state I was in. The sympathetic man immediately gave us a more comfortable room. It was probably through him that the other vacationers learned at what "health resort" I had so recently been an honored guest. No one said a word, for people still refrained from discussing such matters openly. But from the heightened attention, unconcealed sympathy, and even tenderness I encountered at every step, it was easy enough to guess that my story was no longer a secret. Certainly all the attentions lavished on us were not a tribute to my personal charm, though I wish they were, but a manifestation of the Soviet intelligentsia's attitude toward recent events in the country and their victims. All this created a warm atmosphere,

contributing to my inner contentment and mental equili-
brium—even spiritual rejuvenation. One of the vacationers was
a radio announcer, a lively lady who lifted the taboo by telling
over the radio who I was and what I had gone through. This
had a liberating effect on the others and removed all camouflage
from their sympathy for me and my wife. People longed to
throw off the mental oppression they had been living with for
so long. Yet some prejudices and cruel, absurd conventions
were deeply ingrained in their minds, as hard to remove as a
tattoo.

I remember mentioning a noted linguist in a conversation
with an elderly couple who were both doctors of philosophy
and had been affected directly by Stalin's *Marxism and Lin-
guistics*, one of the masterworks penned by that "greatest genius
of all times and nations." In all seriousness they regretted that
my linguist friend "had a dark spot on his biography." I was
surprised, expecting to hear of some dishonest action on his
part, and asked them what they meant. "He has some relative
living abroad," they explained. They could not understand my
vehement reaction to that remark and remained convinced that
having a relative living abroad was compromising enough to
spoil an otherwise spotless life. Yet it was sufficient reason for
me to stay away from such tattooed individuals, despite their
eagerness to be friendly.

In Sochi I played a rather nasty joke on my friend Gelstein,
who was not staying at the same sanatorium but in a nearby
hotel. One day when I came to see him, I found him taking a
shower. I knocked on the bathroom door and shouted in an
authoritative voice: "Gelstein, out for interrogation!" Gelstein
appeared at the door, deathly pale and frightened. I regretted
my prank that very instant. I had not made an allowance for his
prisoner's reflexes. But the episode showed how deep-seated in
our minds was the expectation of a reversal in fortune. We
lacked faith in the altered political situation in the country and
conviction that it would last. That little incident was highly

indicative of the typical psychological pattern of the time—the instinctive fear of the rabbit facing the boa constrictor.

At the health resort I received a letter from Didenko, director of my institute. He wrote in detail about the situation there, the veiled resistance to the new trends among the institute's party members, their unwillingness to reorient thinking that had been dominated for so long by Stalinist norms. Didenko was attempting to prepare me for what awaited me on my return and for the need to put up a struggle against it, in his interests and my own. Frankly, I was too exhausted for more struggle. I longed for peace and quiet after my ordeals, but the situation was not conducive to that.

Didenko told me in his letter how, after my arrest, my fellow party members had been instructed to set up a commission to inspect my laboratory and discover evidence of the sabotage I had been allegedly engaged in. The commission set forth its conclusions in a document approved at the party meeting. Didenko advised me to demand that I be told of its contents and to insist upon its repeal. I couldn't have cared less about that document after I had been rehabilitated by the higher authorities and had my party membership restored. But this repeal was necessary for Didenko, who had been accused of supporting an enemy of the people. Didenko's case was suspended temporarily, but its complete dismissal could only follow my rehabilitation at the local level. So Didenko had a point, which I, in my innocence of party bureaucracy, had not considered.

Upon returning from my vacation, I applied to the institute's party organization, demanding to see whatever documents had been put through in my absence. I requested that these decisions should be either abolished or reconsidered in my presence. I rather expected the party leaders automatically to cancel their decisions. But it was naive to suppose that the fact of my rehabilitation would annul the other accusations. Little did I realize that Stalin's party machine was still functioning and was not going to give way easily. The institute's party leadership,

207

after consulting the district committee, announced that the decisions could not be annulled but were to be reconsidered in my presence. Moreover, our party leadership had apparently been instructed to confirm all the points that had been used to incriminate me, that is, to validate their objectivity. This phenomenon was indicative of an interesting paradox of those days: while the higher governmental and party bodies were willing to disavow the MGB's reputation for infallibility, the local authorities defended their own reputations tooth and nail, maintaining a myth of ethics in which no one believed any longer. My case was not the only one. Right after Stalin's death, cases of resistance to rehabilitation of the innocently accused were quite frequent.

So the Doctors' Plot did not end once and for all in Lubyanka. For me it had a sequel in the party organization of the Tarasevich Institute. The following Friday, the party bureau convened to consider my demand. The document summing up the inspection of my laboratory was read aloud. The gist of the matter was preceded by a long introduction including many biographical particulars: "The Commission consisting of [names of the three members], on the instruction of the Party bureau, has inspected the laboratory of pathologic morphology formerly headed by Professor Yakov Lvovich Rapoport, D.Sc. (Med.), born 1898, a Jew, on the staff of the Institute since 1947." This was followed by a list of faults discovered by the commission that might be classed as sabotage. I don't remember all the details precisely, for most of the accusations were deplorably insubstantial. The commission had little knowledge of pathologic morphology and was not competent to form any sort of opinion about my research, to say nothing of establishing its allegedly harmful nature. All the accusations in the document were contrived and inconclusive, related to minor points and superficial aspects. None of this evidence was worth a bean. But the party bureau had to make do with what was at hand. They discussed the "indictment" point by point, and on each point they pronounced me guilty. The central part of the document—their trump card—concerned personnel: I was accused of sabotage in matters of training. The latter point calls for some clarification.

One of the two "personnel" in my charge at the time was a graduate student whose research I was supervising. She was lazy by nature and had married recently; in the second year of her graduate course, she became pregnant and lost interest in her thesis. I must give her some credit: she sympathized with me over the events of 1952–53, but she was not worried in the least about the end result of her research project. She was well aware of the political situation in the country and knew that I would do my best to ensure that she complete her thesis successfully, in order to avoid being accused of intentionally neglecting a graduate student of Russian nationality. From the moment the campaign against cosmopolitanism was unleashed, such cases became the object of close attention and were sometimes reported—in a biased light—in the press. My student was not mistaken. I had to go against my principles as scientific supervisor and help her complete the thesis she was supposed to defend in the summer of 1953. I wrote many pages of the draft myself and later made numerous corrections and additions to her final copy.

So I was astonished to read in the party indictment that not only had I neglected my duties as scientific supervisor but had not even read this student's thesis. It should be noted that I was the only specialist in pathologic morphology at the institute who could help her, inadequate as she was, in this particular subject. I was so enraged at this point that I demanded that my former student be called in. They complied, and she was summoned. Judging from the woman's confused look, she was not quite prepared for such a confrontation. When the chairman asked her if she confirmed the accusation concerning her thesis, her eyes filled with tears, and through her sobs she confirmed everything without once glancing in my direction. Then I asked her to bring in the draft of her thesis, which bore my numerous corrections and additions to say nothing of many pages written in my hand. Still sobbing, she replied that she had no drafts, her husband had burned them. This seemed so improbable that in different circumstances she would have been quickly exposed as a liar. I had kept all my own drafts, even of early papers, although by that time I had nearly one hundred publications to my name. But she was claiming to have burned her first and only work, which was not even completed. (Later the "burned draft" was found.) None of this could convince my judges. According to the scenario, they were supposed to believe all accusations against me, and they followed this rule to the letter. Then I demanded that the woman present the revised version of her thesis, which also bore many of my penciled annotations. But she said she had left it at her dacha.

The proceedings were adjourned until Monday, but the atmosphere of the trial left me no hope for a favorable outcome. It turned out that in the revised draft all my pencil marks had been erased, although imprints were clearly visible; even an inexperienced investigator could easily establish that the erased marks belonged to me. I was no longer surprised when my former student gave me the cold shoulder on my return to the institute, although she still needed help to finish her thesis and get it defended. In my absence she must have officially dissociated herself from me as scientific supervisor, in order to save her thesis. This was nothing unusual in those cruel days. Children often dissociated themselves from arrested parents, wives from husbands, and close relatives disowned one another to save themselves. Yet most people bore no grudges. The man whose dacha was next to mine was an eminent medical scientist arrested as one of the killer doctors. His former assistant, who held a chair at an affiliated institute, was called upon to denounce his teacher at a meeting devoted to the exposure of the Doctors' Plot. He condemned the doctor forcefully and in the end exclaimed: "I wish I could strangle the scoundrel with my own hands!" Knowing of this incident, I was surprised later to see the potential executioner among my neighbor's guests. I asked if he knew that his guest had publicly denounced him. Of course he knew. "But he couldn't help it," he added. In those vile times, people pardoned treachery, and only a few had enough courage to avoid committing it. As for me, I could never overcome my aversion to any kind of betrayal.

I should note here that meetings denouncing the Doctors' Plot were held in all medical establishments and medical societies. Many doctors and noted medical scientists were asked publicly to denounce their colleagues, and they did, often demanding the death penalty for their close friends. There was one such meeting at the Academy of Medical Sciences. The killer doctors included two members of the Academy: Miron Vovsi and Vladimir Vinogradov (subsequently four more academicians were arrested). The speakers blazed forth with hatred for the accused. Particularly vehement was Zilov, chief of personnel at the academy, who heaped vile antisemitic epithets on the "Zionist" Vovsi. The only person who had the courage to protest (a feat of valor in those times) was Georgy Speransky, the well-known scholar and pediatrician. Still the meeting adopted the resolution it was expected to adopt, in both wording and content.

At the Therapeutists' Society, this social function of denigration was performed by its president, the energetic academician Alexander Myasnikov, a nonparty member and a noted scientist. That academic abused the arrested professors not only as political criminals but also as pseudo-scientists and professional incompetents. Among those he attacked was his friend Miron Vovsi, which did not prevent them from resuming their friendship when things quieted down. Vinogradov was less charitable. He could not forgive either Myasnikov or the professors appointed to give expert opinion in the doctors' case, forgetting that he himself gave an expert opinion in the earlier case of Pletnyov which was far from favorable for the accused.

To come back to my own case, I decided to have nothing more to do with this humiliating "reconsideration." So when the technical secretary of the institute's party bureau came to invite me to another conference the next Monday, I handed her a short written statement: "My experience of attempting to defend my work in the laboratory has convinced me that the present reconsideration is being carried out in the same spirit as the inspection conducted in my absence, during my unlawful arrest. Therefore I refuse to take any part in the revision of the document, which contains nothing but lies. I do not object if this is done in my absence."

There was no answer to my letter, and I considered the matter closed—the form of the closure was all the same to me. Meanwhile I did everything necessary to get the graduate student through to a successful defense of her thesis. Had I followed my natural inclination and refused to do it, she could never have completed the thesis, much less defend it, and so the huge army of holders of advanced medical degrees would have been lacking one cipher. But spite is a poor counsel. Moreover, I realized that my refusal to help her might rebound: it would confirm how unfortunate she was in her scientific supervisor. I do not name her here, for I feel nothing but pity for her.

On the day of the defense (which was held not at our institute but at the Academy of Medical Sciences), the whole party leadership of the institute attended, although the aspiring candidate was not a party member. The defense procedure was routine: the author of the thesis made a report, followed by challengers who commented on various aspects of the paper. In her reply, the author of the thesis thanked her critics for their valuable advice and promised to take it into account in future work. In conclusion she expressed gratitude to her scientific supervisor for his uninterrupted guidance and help (denied at the sitting of the party bureau), and by unanimous vote the academic degree was conferred on her. Soon after, she took a job at another institute, and I lost sight of her.

As the days of Stalin's tyranny receded into the past, the thaw in Soviet society spread, penetrating the minds and everyday lives of the people. Ryumin, the MGB man responsible for fabricating the Doctors' Plot, was shot. I learned of this on the commuter train on the way home from my dacha. A teenage girl sitting opposite me with her mother was reading the morning paper and said: "They shot the man who was torturing the doctors." The announcement went as follows:

At the Supreme Court of the USSR: On July 2–7, 1954, the Military Collegium of the Supreme Court of the USSR held proceedings against M. D. Ryumin, accused of a crime classified under Article 58.7 of the Criminal Code of the RSFSR.

It has been established by the investigation that in the course of his work in the capacity of senior investigator and subsequently chief of the investigation department for special cases at the former Ministry of State Security of the USSR, Ryumin acted as a concealed enemy of the state, in his own careerist and adventurist interests. He fabricated evidence that gave rise to falsified cases involving unlawful arrests of Soviet citizens, including noted figures in the medical profession.

According to the evidence presented by the witnesses for the prosecution, Ryumin resorted to methods prohibited by Soviet law to extract admissions of the gravest of crimes, such as treason, sabotage, and espionage, and also false evidence incriminating innocent persons.

Later investigation revealed the complete groundlessness of these charges. The persons thus accused have now been fully rehabilitated.

Taking into account the special gravity of Ryumin's criminal activities and the harmful consequences of the crimes he committed, the Military Collegium of the Supreme Court of the USSR has sentenced Ryumin to capital punishment—death by shooting.

The sentence has been carried out.

Guilty of numerous innocent deaths, Ryumin finally met his downfall in connection with the Doctors' Plot. He was only one of masses of scoundrels, some of whom were in much higher positions. But only a few of them received their just due (Beria and his henchmen were shot). The announcement of Ryumin's execution was another piece of evidence indicating that the closing of the doctors' case marked the beginning of a serious restructuring of the Soviet system.

And yet the fresh wind seemed not to reach the stagnant party organization at my institute, with its Stalinist notions rigidified in narrow minds. Several weeks later, I was approached again by the secretary of our institute's party organization, Tebyakina, who insisted that we finish the reconsideration of the inspection document. I said I was not at all interested. Tebyakina replied that my letter was a "slap in the face" of the party organization. This argument rather surprised me. After all, I already had a pardon from the supreme judges of political loyalty, which allowed me a certain independence and freedom of criticism. I had no wish to take any part in the comedy of reconsideration and told the secretary that although I did not exactly mean it as a slap in the face, now that she mentioned it, she was probably not far from wrong. Tebyakina assured me that at the recent defense of my graduate student's thesis, their eyes had been opened and now everything would be different. So I agreed to attend the next sitting of our party bureau.

In an atmosphere of overdone friendliness, the session again opened with the reading of the inspection document, including all the biographical details: "The Commission consisting of . . . has examined . . . and established . . . that Professor Yakov Lvovich Rapoport, D.Sc. (Med.), a Jew, etc." This was followed by an enumeration of all the charges one by one. They were unable to close the matter without going into the details once more and canceling each as irrelevant and inconclusive. When it came to my student's thesis, the deputy secretary said that the party organization had been misled on that point by the young woman and suggested that this be included in the minutes. I had been silent until then, but at this point I couldn't help noting that such an excuse would discredit the party organization, which had been misled so easily by a silly young woman who was not even a party member. After they were through reviewing the document, they decided to read what was left of it and, apart from the biographical introduction and the signatures of the commission members, nothing remained. I could not suppress my laughter and said that, in this form, I would sign it. This ridiculous product of party bureaucracy can probably still be found in the party archives of the Tarasevich Institute.

For me, that party meeting was the final curtain in the Doctors' Plot tragedy, which had come down on a farce.

– 10 –

Stalin's Fury

THE READER is probably expecting a logical explanation of how the Doctors' Plot could happen. But I do not consider myself sufficiently qualified to provide an exhaustive analysis of its causes. This could only be done by a professional historian-cum-sociologist with access to all the archives of the Stalin period and those immediately preceding and following it. In other words, this episode can be understood only within a larger context. In my opinion, however, no amount of official documents, even if all were preserved by some miracle and were now made available to researchers, can fully reveal the hidden motives behind the plot. These motives cannot be uncovered until that complex tangle of provocations, intrigues, and struggles within the ruling elite, where defeat meant death, is unraveled. All tyrannies are essentially alike. The tyrant's arbitrary rule is his only logic, and his decisions are often prompted by his entourage, whether he knows it or not.

Stalin's rule was a pure form of tyranny and he himself, the consummate tyrant. Like any autocrat, he was not immune to lesser human weaknesses. Drawing a full psychological portrait of Stalin is a task yet to be accomplished. Many writers have tried their hand, but Stalin's image remains elusive and partial. Since I am by no means a professional investigator but merely a chronicler of events I personally witnessed, I will not attempt to make any contribution to psychological portrait painting. Yet I suspect that the portrait of Stalin is considerably simpler than many people believe and that it falls into a particular type. Stalin's salient features were hypocrisy and perfidy combined with raw cunning (he could catch even wise old birds with chaff); unbridled cruelty and a thirst for blood; the irrational suspiciousness of a paranoic; and considerable physical coward-ice—in short, all the indispensable traits of a tyrant. Collec-tively these traits made Stalin an object for criminological psy-chopathology. "Though this be madness, yet there is method in't," said Polonius. Yet it is a thankless task to search for meth-od and logic in Stalin's actions. Normal human criteria are inapplicable here. Stalin succeeded in introducing his own kind of method into the system ushered in by the Revolution of 1917.

The Doctors' Plot was the logical culmination of Stalin's en-tire illogical system. It defies common sense—all one can do is attempt to analyze the series of events that led up to it. The factual material at our disposal is not only scarce but unreliable. Some of the facts came to light at the Twentieth Party Congress in 1956, while others reached us from semiofficial sources. Col-lectively, they suggest the following picture.

Stalin's personal physician was Vladimir Vinogradov, an ex-cellent clinician of long experience. In his later years, Stalin suffered from hypertension and arteriosclerosis with occasional disturbances in cerebral circulation (he died of a massive cere-bral hemorrhage), which produced multiple small cysts in the brain tissue, particularly in the frontal lobes, as the autopsy revealed. The cysts were the result of the encephalomalacia caused by hypertension and arteriosclerosis. These defects (and especially their localization in the frontal cerebral areas, which are responsible for the complex forms of behavior) and the mental disturbances they brought about served to aggravate Stalin's inherently despotic nature. "Bad temper" that gets con-stantly worse, a distressing phenomenon first noted by family members and friends, is frequently the first symptom of developing cerebral arteriosclerosis. One can imagine the effects such a condition could produce in a born oppressor.

The last time Vinogradov examined Stalin (in early 1952), he found a marked worsening of the ruler's health, which he recorded in Stalin's case history along with strict recommendations to observe a prescribed course of medical treatment and to retire from all public activity. When Beria reported these recommendations to Stalin, he flew into a terrible rage. How dare that impudent quack cast aspersions on his boundless earthly might! According to Khrushchev, he shouted: "Throw him in chains!"

Doing away with Vinogradov alone could not satisfy Stalin's malicious vindictiveness. "The great leader of the world proletariat" was a man of vast enterprise where it concerned human lives. His criminological views were simple and constant: he saw conspiracies everywhere. Only the number of conspirators and their aims and methods varied. Often he himself invented one plot or another, leaving it to the security apparatus, represented by such villains as Vyshinsky, Krylenko, and Ulrich, to supply the details of the script, which was usually quite elaborate. Having invented a plot, Stalin apparently dismissed it from his mind, and when later it came back to him as an elaborately worked-out case, he would think it had really happened. People carried away by an idea often lose their sense of perspective and start believing in a fiction they themselves have invented. There are numerous examples of such beliefs among scientists who would put their faith in any falsehood if it served to corroborate their theories. Maniacal ideas of this kind coexisted in Stalin along with deliberate calculations to liquidate masses of people whom he perceived as obstacles in his path to absolute power.

A paranoic like Stalin could not have been content to take Vinogradov's action as simply the work of one individual. The twisted logic characteristic of his condition went into play. First, he must have recalled numerous instances of doctors' readiness to serve his political ends at the cost of their professional integrity. The certificate of his wife's death written by doctors who swore that she had died of appendicitis, when in actuality she shot herself, surely came to mind. And then there was Sergey Ordzhonikidze's suicide, which the doctors dutifully recorded as cardioplegia on the death certificate. He could have recalled the medical expertise given in connection with the "murders" of Menzhinsky and Gorky by their physicians. (Those charges and the attending verdict were not officially annulled until 1988.) He might have recalled the servile role of leading medical men in the campaign against academicians Orbeli, Stern, and many others who fell into disfavor with Stalin. The campaign to crown Lepeshinskaya as the queen of Soviet science, incited and directed from above, involved well over one hundred scientists of varying degrees of moral turpitude. He certainly knew about the many doctors employed by the MGB who were responsible for reprehensible actions carried out at the bidding of their superiors.

Stalin was not the first to employ medicine and medical men to help achieve personal and political aims. He was well-read enough to know that in all historical epochs medical men were used by politicians to achieve their aims, often of a criminal nature, or to cover up their crimes. He probably saw no reason to be an exception. Social ethics during and after Stalin's rule still awaits objective and intensive sociological analysis. But even now one can say with a considerable degree of certainty that Soviet society at the time did not universally espouse Marxist-Leninist ethics but was a loose conglomeration of extremely varied ethical stands. Any number of scoundrels could be found to carry out any disgraceful scheme. Such persons could also be found among the academic elite. Suffice it to recall the commission of experts set up to investigate the Doctors' Plot. The enlistment of suitable candidates for vile jobs was easy, since any moral scruples they might have were swept aside by reference to state and party necessities. It reminds me of a young lady of easy virtue who retorted upon being rebuked for loose behavior: "Each to her own devices and her own morals."

Stalin never trusted anyone's allegiance to ideals, despite

what World War II should have taught him, while the organs of state security saw everyone as a potential traitor and conspirator—this thesis was Lubyanka's mainstay. Stalin and his lieutenants did their best to corrupt Soviet society, not realizing that there was a limit to how far this moral degradation could go. This limit was determined by the inborn decency and civic-mindedness of the people. Such decency lived on in many scientists. Note that, in the medical profession, it was precisely the most conscientious doctors who fell victim to Stalin's repressions, people who had been trained by the celebrated physicians of old in the finest traditions of Russian medicine. These doctors were not without fault; they were only human and were probably also affected by Stalinism, but they were all physicians in the best sense of the word, faithful to high medical principles and a sense of mission. In their many decades of honest work, they saved countless lives.

Stalin's world view excluded ethical principles. Intoxicated by his witch hunting, he saw covens in every corner. So his fury, initially directed against Vinogradov alone, soon produced the idea of an extensive medical conspiracy. The apparatus of the MGB, headed by Abakumov and after him by Ignatyev, was immediately set into motion. The Doctors' Plot offered unprecedented scope because it concerned Stalin personally. The MGB promptly set about concocting the case according to the usual pattern. They drew up a broad panorama, this time involving the country's leading medical scientists pitted against Soviet statesmen. The general plan was gradually elaborated as details were filled in and specific people were implicated. The first to be arrested were the leading doctors at the Kremlin Hospital, where the MGB recruited Lydia Timashuk, an EKG specialist, to supply them with incriminating information about professors who allegedly prescribed incorrect treatments and gave incorrect medical conclusions. The arrested professors confessed to their crimes under pressure, and Timashuk was proclaimed a heroine. There is no need to remind the reader by what methods such confessions were wrenched from the victims. These tried and true methods had been employed since 1936 and have been described at length in fiction. They included both physical torture and powerful psychological pressure, such as few people could resist.

Initially, the Doctors' Plot had no nationalistic coloring; both Russian and Jewish doctors were implicated. But before long, it was given an antisemitic slant. Ryumin of the MGB was responsible for turning it into a Jewish conspiracy. According to Khrushchev, Ryumin informed Stalin that there existed a "Jewish bourgeois nationalist conspiracy" in the pay of the American intelligence service, and that State Security Minister Abakumov was aware of it from the information supposedly supplied by previously arrested Yakov Etinger. Wishing to conceal this from Stalin (why he should want to do that is a mystery), he had ordered Etinger killed in prison. The real cause of Etinger's death will probably never be established. In his later years, he suffered from coronary sclerosis with frequent attacks of angina pectoris, and most probably the ordeals he underwent were simply too much for his heart. Stalin gave Ryumin's information full credence. Abakumov was removed from his post and arrested (replaced by I. D. Ignatyev), and Ryumin was entrusted with full control of the doctors' case. Thus one spider devoured another. Ryumin was diligently developing this case in the required direction when he was cut short by Stalin's death. Soon after, Ryumin was shot for his role in the plot. Later, Abakumov and some other active MGB officers were tried in open court and sentenced to death as well.

This is only a glimpse through the backdoor of Stalin's charnel house, compared with which the horrors of the Spanish Inquisition are mere child's play.

Postscript, 1988

THIRTY-FIVE YEARS have passed since the doctors' case was closed. Recollections of those events gradually fade from people's memories, leaving only a general impression of terror and helplessness. The emotional excitement that moved my pen as I wrote this book has subsided, but it is not altogether gone.

Now and then vicious attacks are made on the medical profession, which revive memories of the Doctors' Plot. I know it for a fact. Somewhere in the dark depths of our society lurk forces that are prepared to use the same foul means for their own ends. They are only waiting for an opportunity. Well, they are waiting in vain! I am convinced of it, and my conviction rests on the historical changes that have been wrought in the entire structure of Soviet society by perestroika and the new thinking.

One reason for my optimism is the fate of this book. I started writing it in the 1970s, with no hope of ever seeing it published. The sociopolitical climate was not yet ripe for that. But I felt compelled to leave a literary testimony of the Doctors' Plot, in expectation of the time—which I was sure would come eventually—when reason would triumph over prejudice and my manuscript would reach the reading public. This time has now come. I have lived to see it, and I am happy. I often quote some lines from Tyutchev's poem "Cicero":

> O blessed is the man who lives
> When earth's own fate must be decided!
> To dine with gods he is invited
> And counsel at their table gives.

May the survivors of those evil times be consoled by these verses, which can help them come to terms with the past.

Acknowledgments on behalf of my father, Yakov Rapoport

The idea to publish my father's book in the United States came to me one summer's day in 1986. I was enjoying a Chagall painting at the Budapest Museum of Fine Arts when I had the good fortune of meeting two Americans: Frances and Morton Clurman. We became fast friends, and I entrusted them with the secret of my father's manuscript. We had been hiding the manuscript in the Soviet Union for more than ten years without hope of publishing it. The Clurmans were very sympathetic, and this meeting played a decisive role in the future life of my family.

Meanwhile the situation in the Soviet Union changed drastically. Thanks to Mikhail Gorbachev's changes in policy, the book was published in the USSR in December 1988 and became a bestseller.

Russian version in hand, I came to America at the invitation of the Clurmans. They introduced me to their friends Leonard and Elky Shatzkin, who in turn recommended me to the agent Lynn C. Franklin. With Lynn's extraordinary dedication, we were able to introduce this book into western countries. I cannot thank this wonderful woman enough for all that she has done.

The book was translated into English in the Soviet Union by

Natalya Perova and Raisa Bobrova, who had their work cut out for them.

My short memoir, included as the prologue to the book, was translated into English with the help of the Englishman Dan Richardson and the American Eric Whitlock. Eric spent many hours with me, working devotedly. My childish verses were translated by Gil Peterson. Our translation was then edited by Susan Schapiro and Elizabeth McKeon. We are grateful to our publishers and all of our friends for their invaluable help.

N.R.

EARLY PLOTTERS

PROFESSOR VASILY TERNOVSKY headed the department of anatomy at the Kazan Medical Institute before World War II. He was
elected a member of the Soviet Academy of Medical Sciences when it
was set up. Ternovsky moved from Kazan to Moscow and was appointed head of the department of anatomy at the Second Medical
Institute and also head of the division of normal anatomy at the newly
formed Institute of Morphology of the Academy of Medical Sciences.
These posts were, in fact, far in excess of his merits.

A personnel department chief I once knew, while composing a
character reference for an employee and noting his high level of professional competence, added: "but his external appearance does not
correspond to the post he holds." God knows what he meant by that
digression, but, as regards Ternovsky, one had to admit that his external appearance fully corresponded to all the posts he held. He could
have easily served as the model for a stylized scientist, artist, or
orchestra conductor: an aquiline nose on a lean, clean-shaven face,
adorned by a pair of gold-rimmed spectacles; fine hair carefully
combed back from a rather low forehead; never a trace of a smile on
his face and hence an expression of deep thoughtfulness. He wore a
blue beret instead of a hat, another artistic touch. Ternovsky spoke
slowly, using turns of speech characteristic of prerevolutionary intellectuals. At his lectures the dry matter-of-fact subject of anatomy was
presented as a dramatic recitation. His usual greeting to the students
was "Dear friends," a demagogic device designed to express the lofty
indulgence of a distinguished scientist toward youthful listeners. He

would poetize anatomical terms effusively: "Listen to how fine it sounds: *protuberantia occipitalis magna!*"—much like the character in Chekhov who delighted in the beauty of Greek words: "Anthropos!" But this pomposity concealed vacuity and a very superficial knowledge of his subject. Perhaps he had known anatomy at one time, but had forgotten much of it—a fact that became immediately obvious in even a brief professional discussion with the man. It was just as clear from some of his actions.

I came into close contact with Ternovsky at the Institute of Morphology where I was deputy director for research. Ternovsky was head of the division of normal anatomy, and he had a staff of twenty-four. Since the institute did not have suitable premises, such as an autopsy theater, a cold storage room, and such, the division was located in the anatomy department of the Second Medical Institute (where Ternovsky was also a professor). It was in fact an overgrown appendix of that department and received financial support from it; the majority of the staff members combined work in Ternovsky's division and in the Second Medical Institute. The job of coordinating all these activities was fully entrusted to Ternovsky, whose main concern was the enlargement of his personal income. Although he seemed well taken care of with his two high salaries, plus the fee he received as member of the Academy of Medical Sciences, he could not resist the temptation to pull off some very shady deals involving the anatomy library.

He was also caught red-handed in criminal plagiarism when Medgiz Publishers brought out a *Manual of Anatomical Technique* supposedly authored by Ternovsky, but which was in fact a translation from the German of a supplement to an anatomy textbook. Ironically, the author of the textbook did not include the supplement in his second edition because, as he noted in the foreword, he did not think it good enough. Ternovsky apparently hoped that Soviet anatomists would know the second edition and forget about the supplement to the first. But he miscalculated. The meticulous Pyotr Dyakonov discovered the plagiarism and publicized it far and wide. Ternovsky's sole contribution to the manual were some crude anatomical drawings, which often testified to their author's gross ignorance. For instance, he represented the patella, which is an independent anatomical detail, as part of the femur.

There was a great to-do, which even found reflection in the press.

But Ternovsky's high-ranking friends at once set about whitewashing him, and in this they were fully successful. The blame was shifted onto Ternovsky's anonymous assistants (nobody was punished, since no names were given), who had allegedly abused the trust of their chief.

As for research, which the division of anatomy was supposed to perform, it was confined to the translation into Russian of a work by the medieval anatomist Vesalius. When the translation was finally published, it was discovered that it had been made not from the Latin original but from a German version. This was yet another fraud, which incidentally cost the state a pretty penny.

Ternovsky had a devoted aide in his scurrilous activities. This was his senior research assistant Sarah Dzugayeva, another typical product of Stalin's epoch. She was an Ossete by nationality, and the Georgian variant of her surname was identical to Stalin's true surname: Dzhugashvili. She made a point of informing all and sundry whose namesake she was, so that they should treat her with the proper awe. After the personality cult was denounced, an attempt was made to fire her: it was well known that she was a useless scientific worker who substituted intrigue for research. But however hard the leaders of the institute tried, and no matter how great their prestige, Dzugayeva was not to be dislodged.

In the fall of 1949, the Institute of Morphology was instructed by the presidium of the academy to reduce its monthly expenses by dismissing unneeded staff members. The decision concerning who was to go rested with the institute's administration, but it was recommended that, rather than weaken laboratories that were doing fruitful work by an equal reduction of personnel in all departments, structural units that were of no particular scientific value would be dissolved entirely. Such, unmistakably, was Ternovsky's division of anatomy. Convinced that it was scientifically sterile and a waste of money to the state, I suggested that it should be disbanded. My idea was supported by the institute's director, Abrikosov, and the academy's presidium endorsed our proposal too.

We should have foreseen the explosive consequences, the reverberations of which reached me for a long time afterward. The first reaction came from head of the academy's personnel department, Zilov, whose mind set was in full accord with Stalin's precepts. When the order concerning the abolition of the anatomy division was issued, he was away from Moscow, and when he came back he was appalled. His original idea had been to reduce the research staff by getting rid of its Jewish members, and the liquidation of Ternovsky's division did nothing to help him achieve this end. But the order had already been signed by the academy's president and could not be revoked, especially since the ostensible purpose of personnel reduction—economizing—had been fully met. Zilov insisted that some Jewish staff members should also be dismissed. In putting forward this demand, he dispensed with the fig leaf altogether. But, without some kind of cover, such an action with respect to competent research scientists would have been too outrageous to attempt. Zilov was in a quandary. So he earmarked two victims whose surnames he found suspicious. But here too he was out of luck. One of the victims proved extremely refractory and put up a gallant opposition to Zilov's plans. Unexpectedly, she gained the support of the mighty Lysenko, who wrote a letter to Abrikosov in which he spoke approvingly of the woman's work (in the field of cancer heredity) and objected to her dismissal. The fact of Lysenko's interference in the affairs of an institute that had nothing to do with him personally is highly characteristic. Another curious aspect of the affair was that the victim adhered to the condemned "Mendelism-Morganism," but, in his ignorance of genetics, Lysenko failed to grasp this. As a result of the intercession, Zilov had to be content with just one victim, who turned out to be only half-Jewish. His antisemitic mountain gave birth to merely half a mouse.

But to get back to Ternovsky. There is a gloomy adage which says that no good deed ever goes unpunished. Well, my deed—good if not for Ternovsky, then for everyone concerned with science—was certainly punished. The punishment as such only came later, but a warning of its coming reached me soon after the anatomy division was disbanded. I was informed of it by a person holding a responsible post at the academy (in strict confidence, of course). I shall cite the first lines of this warning, which was addressed to the all-powerful executioner Lavrenty Beria, the chief of state security: "We deem it necessary to draw your attention to the Institute of Normal and Pathologic Morphology under the Academy of Medical Sciences. The post of director is held by Academician A. I. Abrikosov, but a band of Jewish bourgeois nationalists are active behind his back. The band is headed by Professor Y. L. Rapoport, and its members are [here followed a list of major Jewish scientists]. This gang, under the leadership of

Rapoport and with the connivance of Academician Abrikosov, has liquidated the Institute of Morphology's Anatomy Division, which was headed by an eminent scientist, a member of the Academy of Medical Sciences, Professor V. N. Ternovsky. The Anatomy Division was the best at the Institute—a real gem—which published excellent research materials." And so it continued for two pages, shamelessly extolling the scientific attainments of Ternovsky and stigmatizing the nefarious activities of the "gang."

Beria sent the letter (written undoubtedly by Ternovsky himself) to the presidium of the academy, asking them to send him the pertinent facts. I know nothing of the correspondence that followed, but, judging from the absence of repercussions, the charges must have been disproved convincingly enough by the presidium. Still the letter left a sinister trace, and I was reminded of it in the grim days of 1953.

The "wronged" anatomists did not rest content with this letter. There followed another denunciation, inspired by the same characters and penned by one of my graduate students. The story deserves to be told in greater detail.

Lydia Ishchenko was admitted to graduate courses at the Institute of Morphology in 1948. Her adviser was Director Abrikosov himself, and his laboratory was situated on the premises of the department of pathology of the First Medical Institute, on the lane that is now called Abrikosov. A year later, the director decided that Ishchenko should be dismissed for lack of ability and ill temper—she had quarreled with every single person in the laboratory. The personnel department of the academy, however, decided otherwise and transferred her to my laboratory at the First Gradskaya Hospital, where she was to continue working on her thesis under my supervision. I refused to accept a person with a reputation as an incorrigible squabbler, who had managed to drive to extreme measures even the mild and patient Abrikosov. But my objections were overruled. Moreover, I was given the responsibility of making sure she completed her project and defended her thesis. I wondered at the time what powerful agency was pulling strings on Ishchenko's behalf.

For the first few weeks, she behaved tolerably well, probably pacified by the cooperativeness and good nature of my staff, whom I had urged to avoid conflicts with her. She was obviously a person of little culture; her vocabulary was scant, and she kept away from everybody. She just barely coped with her share of the autopsies and showed neither ability nor inclination for this work. I told her to continue working on the project that Abrikosov had chosen for her thesis and helped her draw up a research plan. She attended the classes in English and political science which were mandatory for all graduate students. All my assistants—everybody who came in contact with her, in fact—believed that she was mentally unbalanced.

During the whole first year at my laboratory she resisted all my attempts to monitor the progress of her research, either postponing the date for a report or simply avoiding me. When she entered the third and final year of graduate study, I made a concerted attack, insisting that I be shown whatever she had done on her thesis. She refused point-blank to show me her histological specimens, with a broad hint that I or somebody else at the laboratory might try to use them for our own ends—in other words, to steal them. Finally she agreed, in response to my persistent badgering, to give me a written report on her work. She told me, by the way, that her thesis was quite ready and that the conclusions had been formulated. When I expressed my surprise that she should have formulated conclusions before the specimens were duly analyzed and arranged, and before the work had been written out, she declared: "Any fool can collect and describe specimens, but not everyone can make good conclusions."

I was staggered. What was I to do? After all, I had been made responsible for seeing that her work was completed in time. When I informed the academy about this state of affairs, they just shrugged the matter off, repeating that Ishchenko must complete her graduate studies without mishap. Again I put the pressure on, demanding to be acquainted at least with her conclusions, and at last she agreed to meet me. On the appointed day (after numerous reminders) she came to my office with a sheaf of papers in her hand, saying that she would read them out to me. I even agreed to that. She began speaking, turning over the sheets, and it was obvious from her manner that she was not reading at all but simply improvising, only pretending to look at her notes. Her improvisations lacked any sense whatever. I managed to catch a glimpse of the front sides of the sheets of paper she was carefully keeping out of my sight (she was holding them fanwise). Some had only a few lines scribbled on top. I could do nothing but demand her expulsion; a graduate student's expulsion so close to the deadline for a thesis defense was unprecedented and reflected on me as her supervisor. Still my patience had been exhausted, and I informed her of this decision.

One fine day, as they say, I got a call from the Institute of Experimental Medicine, where I was informed that a *Pravda* correspondent was making the rounds of the laboratories, asking the staff all kinds of questions, mainly about the person of Rapoport, his participation in the training of scientific personnel, and his attitude toward young researchers and their work. They spoke highly of me, for I had helped budding scientists any way I could, and many of them had done their courses in pathology at my laboratory. The correspondent also asked about Ishchenko and was unanimously informed that she was unbalanced. I went over to the institute toward the end of the day and found that the correspondent was still there; but he showed not the slightest interest in me and did not ask for an interview, although I was the deputy director for research.

The next day, a commission suddenly descended upon my laboratory (I don't remember who its members were—they were all strangers to me). Again they did not ask to see me but questioned my staff as to whether they were satisfied with my supervision of their work, the amount of time I devoted to them, and if I showed any preference for some (Jews in particular) to the detriment of others. They were particularly interested in my relationship with Ishchenko, asked if I had been persecuting her, and made no bones about hoping for a positive answer to this last question. They did not get it and were obviously displeased. I have no doubt that the commission arrived with ready-made conclusions (just as Ishchenko had ready-made conclusions for her nonexistent thesis), and the visit to my laboratory was merely a formality.

The date for the next sitting of the institute's Academic Council, to be chaired by Abrikosov, was approaching. At that sitting, Ishchenko reported on her progress. The *Pravda* correspondent was also there. Ishchenko's speech was painful to hear: a hodge-podge of words jumbled together helter-skelter by an obviously ignorant and not-quite-sane person. The report was voted unsatisfactory. The correspondent, a young man of pleasant appearance, sat in one of the back rows of the auditorium with the younger members of the scientific staff. After the proceedings were closed, somebody asked him what he thought of Ishchenko. He evaded the issue, saying that not everything was clear to him. I ran into him by chance while entering the subway and asked him for his impressions. He would not give me a direct answer but said that he would report to the editor and that an article would probably not be published. At that point, I didn't realize what kind of article he had in mind.

The coin only dropped when I was shown a letter—many pages of typescript—that Ishchenko had sent to *Pravda*. In this denunciatory letter, she wrote that she had made a major scientific discovery that she had to keep secret from me and my staff, for I had made persistent attempts to appropriate it. She wrote in great detail about the persecution she had suffered at my hands because she was not Jewish, persecutions in which all Jewish staff members took part. In a conversation with me about the affair, Vice-President of the Academy Nikolai Ozeretsky, a psychiatrist, said that Ishchenko obviously suffered from a severe form of schizophrenia, and I had been saved by the fact that this became obvious to anyone who spoke to her for five minutes. She was not a suitable candidate for the heroic role of a victim of persecution, or else I would have found myself in very deep water. Then I realized that plans had been made for an article in *Pravda* that would have made mincemeat of me.

As I read the letter of denunciation, I had a feeling that many of its formulations were familiar. I recognized the handwriting, the same as that of the author of the letter to Beria. Then I recalled what my assistants had told me about Ishchenko's strange interest in Ternovsky's division and her frequent visits there, apparently to discuss her work. All that remained unclear was who had put her in touch with Ternovsky and his aide Dzugayeva, for, being so aloof and disoriented, she could have had no idea of their existence.

Many years passed. After Stalin's death, when the doctors' case was dismissed, the political and moral atmosphere in the country began to clear. I had long forgotten the events connected with Lydia Ishchenko, who had vanished into thin air. Suddenly, some ten or twelve years after the incident (which occurred in the spring of 1951), I heard a ring at the door and women's voices in the hall. I was working in my study; it was nearly 8:00 in the evening and quite dark. Our maid told me a woman wanted to see me. I said to let her in and saw none other than Ishchenko. She had become repulsively fat—this is characteristic of mentally ill people who often suffer from metabolic dysfunctions. In her hands she held a tattered file. At first I was startled, even a little frightened, as if I were seeing a ghost. I offered her a chair. She sat down and started repeating the same phrases over and over again: "They will summon you and question you. Here, I've brought these papers so you will know." With that, she pushed across the desk the pages of her letter to *Pravda*, which I had no difficulty in recognizing though they were dog-eared and yellowed with age. I tried to reassure her, saying that nobody would summon me or question me. I insisted that I had no need of the papers, but she kept repeating, "They will summon you, they will question you," and kept pushing that worn record of human baseness toward me. With great difficulty I calmed her, saw her into the hall and out of the apartment, and returned to my study, greatly disturbed by this visitation from the past, by this horrible living ghost. The unfortunate woman had preserved her letter for a decade and finally decided to give it to me as proof of repentance, an act prompted by her morbid schizophrenic conscience. I felt revulsion, but as a victim of the epoch the woman was inexpressibly pitiful.

LINA STERN
Persecution of an Academician

THE NAME OF Lina Solomonovna Stern, member of the Soviet Academy of Sciences and the Medical Academy, is but vaguely known to the modern generation of medical scientists, having been supplanted by new names and discoveries. Her image has been preserved only in the memory of those few of her contemporaries who are still alive, including the author of these pages.

Lina Stern was born into a family of well-to-do Latvian Jews, received a medical education in Switzerland, and upon graduation from Geneva University in 1904 was invited to join the department of physiology at the university, which was then headed by Professor Prevost, a well-known physiologist. Stern soon became Prevost's assistant and won recognition in scientific circles with her work, especially in the field of oxidation enzymes. She presented her papers at major international conferences and congresses and became quite popular in the world of medical science, which was still small enough to allow for extensive personal contacts. The latter were facilitated for Stern by her command of the major European languages. Her friends joked that she could speak all known languages, including Yiddish, but in fact Yiddish was the one language she did not know. In 1917, Stern was made a professor in the department of biochemistry of Geneva University (at the time there was no clear-cut borderline between physiology and biochemistry), and she held this post until she decided to move to the Soviet Union in 1925. She was quite well-off: she earned some 20,000 Swiss francs annually, since, in addition to heading her department, she was also a consultant to a number of pharmaceutical firms. She developed a method of obtaining hormonally active drugs, which she perfected while working in Moscow, used to extract "metabolites" of various organs and tissues. This had to do with implanting tissues in a nutritive medium to which they yielded up the products of their vital activity.

In the final phase of her life in Geneva, Stern undertook the study of the special physiological mechanism in the central nervous system which ensures constancy of the internal medium of the brain, and which protects it from harmful external influences, primarily from substances contained in the blood that may damage the nervous tissue of the brain. She called this mechanism the "hematoencephalic barrier" (that is, a barrier between the blood and the brain tissue), and this term has since become firmly established in medicine and biology. Subsequently she extended the principle of barrier mechanisms, based on the permeability of blood capillaries, to all the organs of the body, and it was christened the "histohematic barrier," a term also used in present-day physiology.

Thus, by the time Lina Stern moved to the Soviet Union, she had made a name for herself in science: she had numerous scientific works to her credit and enjoyed both material and academic prosperity in peaceful bourgeois Geneva. And all this she exchanged without, as she put it, a moment's hesitation (she was generally one to make quick decisions) for a new life in a new environment—that of a society in the throes of building socialism, where peace and quiet were the last things to be expected. There was a streak of "adventurism" in her character, an intuitive thirst for the new. The same applied to her research. Her friends in Geneva and elsewhere in the western world tried to dissuade her from going to Russia: "You will be robbed there, both in the financial and academic sense, and in the end the Cheka will nab you and exile you to Siberia." But these prophecies and the prospect of parting with her friends did not deter her, and she accepted the proposal of her old friends Alexei Bach and Boris Zbarsky to come to the Soviet Union to teach and conduct research. To understand the subsequent events of her life in the Soviet Union, I should outline the academic scene of the 1920s and its relation to the character of Lina Stern.

Ivan Pavlov then reigned supreme in physiology the world over. There is no need to comment on his contribution to science, and in his mother country he was deservedly the indisputable leader in the field.

All of Soviet physiology was Pavlovian physiology; all physiologists who taught and did research at establishments of higher education (in those years science was still concentrated there rather than at research institutes) were in one way or another Pavlov's students and followers. Now this atmosphere of scientific and political unity was invaded by an alien, Lina Stern, and she received a far from amiable reception.

For the sake of objectivity, I must admit that her own character contributed to such a reception. Her appearance was hardly winning, and one who met her for the first time was rarely attracted by her person. She was rather short and stout, had short graying hair, did not have a good command of Russian, and often hesitated in search of the necessary word until her interlocutor prompted her. She spoke with a thick French accent. Her character and, consequently, her actions and relationships with people were contradictory in the extreme, but this very contradictoriness made for a special kind of integrity, for an original and nonstandard makeup.

Lina was often naive in assessing situations and events, and this was paradoxically combined with an astuteness in judgments that bespoke a keen intellect. Her trustfulness was whimsically combined with suspiciousness. The former was often made use of by various scientific scoundrels, who took advantage of her experience and authority for their own nefarious ends; the latter was often directed against her close associates and devoted students. Democratism in relations with her subordinates, simplicity, and accessibility were combined with quirky despotism. Breadth of heart in big matters was combined with utter miserliness in small things. Aggressive bluntness, which was perceived as a complete absence of tact and earned her in a short time quite a few enemies, went side by side on occasion with genuine diplomatic talent. But all this was made up for by a brilliant mind, a sparkling wit, and an absolute dedication to science. This weird medley of positive and negative traits often bred dislike and were used against her by her enemies. Even people close to Stern said that one had to love her very much in order to forgive her great faults.

Lina Stern devoted her entire life to science, sacrificing marriage and having a family. I discovered that this sacrifice had not merely been declarative but had actually taken place. In 1928 I published a paper (one of my first) in a foreign journal. It had to do with a severe complication in malaria, and it attracted the interest of many scientists abroad. I received requests not only for reprints of the article but also for tissue samples. At that time, no difficulties had yet been put in the way of contacts with colleagues abroad, and it was easy enough to comply with these requests. A regular correspondence developed with several colleagues abroad. Among others, I received a letter from the British Professor B., which was not a formal request but a friendly note (relations between scientists at this time were determined not by age, scientific record, and rank, but by interest in one another's work). Lina Stern, entering my study, happened to see the letter on my desk, in an envelope bearing the return address. Seeing the handwriting, she became extremely agitated and pelted me with questions: how had I come to know B. and what did he write to me about? Some time later she told me why the sight of the letter had agitated her so much. B. had been the only serious love in her life and they were engaged to be married. But her fiancé, who adhered to the traditional English view of the family and the function of a wife, explained that he expected her, once married, to discontinue her scientific career. Lina broke off the engagement. The marriage never took place, but both of them remained true to their love and neither married. They met during her frequent trips abroad in the initial period of her life in the Soviet Union; I have reason to believe that she went abroad for the express purpose of seeing him. This apparently was the only romance in Lina's life. She did not shy away from the theme in friendly chats, but invariably made a joke of it. Yet I suspect that this jocular manner was a guise for heartache (not perceived as such or, perhaps, consciously suppressed) and a yearning for a full life. Though she was a scientist of very high standing, Lina Stern never stopped being a woman.

Having subordinated her personal life to science, Stern was often intolerant toward her female assistants, who combined research with duties as wives and mothers. When she selected her staff, her guiding principle was to draw women into science. Today women researchers are so common that Stern's preoccupation with the idea may seem outdated. But things were very different in the 1920s and 1930s. Women were engaged in a struggle for the right to take part in the various endeavors of public life, a struggle begun by the suffragettes. So special efforts were needed to foster every woman researcher. And wherever a staff member was distracted from scientific work by the demands of his or her family (the birth of a child, children's illness, various other household duties), Stern resented this "betrayal" of science and responded to it violently, sometimes in insulting terms. She absolutely refused to take account of the difficult everyday life of her women assistants and would not listen to their explanations. This undoubtedly was an expression of egocentrism on the part of an individual unburdened by a family, comfortably off, and free of attachments. Stern had little affection to spare even her own relatives.

Stern's conflict with her physiologist colleagues began immediately upon her arrival in the Soviet Union. No doubt she was hard to get along with, but another problem was that she had difficulty taking her bearings in an academic milieu that was new to her and gave her an unfriendly reception. When she set about organizing work at the department of physiology in the Moscow Second University (later the medical department of this university was made into the Second Medical Institute), she had to start practically from scratch, selecting research personnel, obtaining equipment, fixing up the premises to suit her needs, and organizing courses that were to include a large number of lab demonstrations and independent experiments. The task was really herculean, and it required all of Stern's indomitable energy and the support of her few but influential friends to set the teaching process into motion and to train the staff she had recruited. This training included elementary methods of physiological experimentation, beginning with tying the experimental animal to the table, making subcutaneous, intravenous, and intracerebral injections, and ending with complicated manipulations. Stern set great store by every member of her staff and spared no effort on their practical and theoretical training, to the point of staying overnight in the laboratory if the work demanded it.

It was for this reason that she never forgot the tragic story of her graduate student K. The victim was a pleasant and gifted young man, who was married to a beautiful but not particularly virtuous woman. She began an affair with a young scientist, who eventually became a member of the academy. Her husband K. was so broken up by her infidelity that he committed suicide, taking an overdose of chloral hydrate. Stern retained inimical feelings for the academician for the rest of her life, and their relations were extremely strained. When once I told her that she was doing harm to herself by nursing that long-standing grudge, she replied that it was not in her nature to nurse grudges but that she could not forget. In actual fact, vindictiveness was quite in her nature.

Despite all the difficulties, work at her department eventually got underway. The central theme was the hematoencephalic barrier. I also had something to do with this research and had some violent conflicts with Stern because of our different approaches to specific aspects of the problem. She did not seem to mind these clashes, and I think she even approved of my scientific temperament. But yet another conflict resulted in a complete break between us. We never worked together after that, though we remained friends to the end of her life, with a few short-lived quarrels, again due to our explosive temperaments. I still have the first, 1935, edition of the research papers written at her institute, one of them my own. The book bears the following inscription in Stern's hand: "To my friend Yakov Lvovich, as a memento of our struggle and friendship."

Until the mid-thirties, Stern went abroad almost every year to attend international conferences and to maintain personal contacts with her colleagues (all this was later presented as incriminating evidence against her). Many of her foreign colleagues came to her laboratory, bringing along complicated apparatus for special investigations and training her staff to use it. This contributed greatly to the success of their research.

In 1925, Vladimir Zelenin, an eminent internist, founded the Medical and Biological Research Institute under the auspices of Glavnauka (Chief Directorate of Scientific Establishments), which was headed by Fyodor Petrov, a veteran communist and associate of Lenin. This institute was envisaged by its sponsors as a complex of therapeutical (mainly cardiological) clinics and experimental laboratories. It was the embryo of the future Academy of Medical Sciences. The central clinic of the institute, which was initially based at the Novo-Ekaterininskaya Hospital, was headed by Zelenin himself. The experimental laboratories grouped around it were headed by Alexander Bogomolets (subsequently president of the Ukrainian Academy of Sciences); Alexei Kulyabko, who went down in medical science as the first experimenter to restore the activity of a heart removed from a corpse (a child's) by passing a salt through it; Mark Sereisky, a well-known psychiatrist and biochemist; and Lina Stern. This institute trained such famous scientists as Nikolai Sirotinin, Miron Vovsi, Lazar Vogelson, Boris Kogan, and Nina Medvedeva. Before long, however, the Medical and Biological Institute became a target for attacks from without, lost its initial substance, and in the early thirties

239

was reorganized into the Medical and Genetic Institute, headed by Solomon Levit, the pioneer of medical genetics in the Soviet Union, who later (in 1938) was arrested and shot. When the Medical and Biological Institute was reorganized, Stern, thanks to the support of Petrov, preserved her laboratory within the system of Glavnauka and subsequently reorganized it into the Institute of Physiology under the auspices of the Academy of Sciences. In 1938 she became the first woman to be elected to the academy in the Soviet Union (and in the world as well). A book about the famous women of Europe (*Fuhrende Frauen Europas*), published in Germany, allotted considerable space to her.

I do not intend to give a detailed chronicle of Lina Stern's life but merely to outline the path that ended in an attempt to destroy her— scientifically and physically—as a particular social phenomenon that was characteristic of the postwar period of the Stalin era. So, while omitting many details of her biography, I must mention her reaction to the rapprochement between the Soviet Union and Nazi Germany, which was marked among other things by Ribbentrop's visit to Moscow in 1939. Stern reacted to these developments with pain and shock; she believed they undermined the principles of the Soviet system (she had joined the Communist Party of the Soviet Union in 1930) and increased the threat that Nazism would spread beyond the boundaries of Germany. When a major statesman tried to explain to her that the rapprochement with Germany was "a marriage of convenience," she retorted: "Even a marriage of convenience produces children, but I can't imagine what kind of children this particular marriage will produce!" This was a farsighted prophecy.

World War II began with Hitler's attack on Poland, which was soon followed by our own invasion of Finland. In this war, the method of treating traumatic shock was developed at Lina Stern's institute and under her direction was subjected to its first practical tests. Theoretically, the method was based on her teaching of the hematoencephalic barrier, which not only protected the nervous centers from various harmful substances contained in the blood, but also barred the way to these centers for medicinal substances injected to restore the normal functioning of the brain following various lesions. In this way, the idea was born (not absolutely new) about the need to find healing substances that would act directly on the nervous centers, bypassing the hematoencephalic barrier, of which the main structural elements were the walls of the capillaries and precapillaries. It was suggested that the hematoencephalic barrier could be circumvented by introducing the medical preparation directly into the spinal fluid, which washes all cells of the brain. The preparation was injected into the cerebello-medullary cistern containing this fluid, which is situated beneath the occipital lobes of the brain. Many disputed the theoretical foundation of the method, basing their arguments on the anatomy of the brain and the manner in which the spinal fluid flows within it. When used during the Finnish war in cases of shock, the method often proved effective. To propagate it, Stern even made a trip to the frontline.

Soon after, Nazi Germany attacked the Soviet Union. Traumatic shock was widespread among the wounded. Attempts were made to publicize treating it with injections into the cerebello-medullary cistern of the brain, but the method was not widely applied—either because it required sophisticated surgical techniques or because the results were contradictory. At any rate, this method did not receive the support of the head of the Medical Board of the Soviet Army, Efim Smirnov (Minister of Health of the USSR after the war), and the chief surgeon of the Soviet Army, Nikolai Burdenko. I cannot agree with Stern, who on a number of occasions alleged that her method had been intentionally ignored by these people.

When Stern's institute, which had been evacuated to Alma-Ata in 1941, returned to Moscow in 1943, she continued the efforts to have her method accepted to fight various diseases, even those like alimentary dystrophy, and particularly specific diseases of the nervous system (viral and other encephalites, tubercular meningitis, and so on). Here chance came to her aid, as often happens not only in medicine.

A girl of ten, Ira, contracted tubercular meningitis. At that time (in 1946) the illness was totally lethal—no cases of recovery were known. In the United States, a new antibiotic, streptomycin, had just been developed, the second after penicillin. It possessed a broad spectrum of antibacterial action and, specifically, was very effective against the pathogen of tuberculosis—Koch's bacillus. The antibiotic had already found extensive clinical application in the treatment of tuberculosis and had come to play an important role in controlling this dread disease. Ira's parents had found out about Lina Stern's method, and they also had information about the antibiotic developed in the United States. So they approached Stern with the request that she cure their daughter using her method. Stern arranged to have some streptomycin sent to her very quickly (it was on the list of "strategic" materials and could be exported only by special permission of the U.S. Congress), and treatment was started under her direction. Streptomycin was injected into the cerebello-medullary cistern of the brain. The girl recovered from tubercular meningitis, although she did not escape deafness, caused by the specifically toxic action of streptomycin on the auditory nerves.

This was the first case of recovery from tubercular meningitis (at least in the Soviet Union) and was perceived as a miracle. The method thus attracted general interest. A special conference was held, and the participants reported their observations of the method's efficacy in different diseases. Most of the speakers were from the Institute of Physiology, and this undoubtedly biased their conclusions about the clinical effectiveness of the method. Not that anyone was deliberately misrepresenting facts and exaggerating results, but the proponents of the method suffered, on the one hand, from an excess of enthusiasm and, on the other, from insufficient information—only natural in the case of experimental physiologists—about the pathology of disease in its natural course and in one method of treatment or another. There have been many such instances in the history of medicine when the developer, under the experimental conditions of a particular treatment—physiological, bacteriological, whatever—ventured personally to assess its effectiveness in practice, that is, when tested on patients. Illness is a complicated process that has its own laws of development, with a specific beginning, sequel, and conclusion. Only a practicing physician knows these laws, for he sees their manifestations in his everyday work; he takes cognizance of them and tries to use them to direct the course of the illness toward recovery. And only a practicing physician can be the final judge of the curative value of a particular medicine or method. There have been countless conflicts between the developer of a method and those who tested it on patients. There were also numerous conflicts between Stern and those who tested her method in clinical conditions. But at that time I am writing about, any event, despite its content and actual significance, could acquire political overtones, often with a fatal ending for the source.

The attempts of Stern to have her method widely accepted gradually acquired political overtones. Not all was clear from a scientific point of view. Some specialists maintained that there was no need to introduce streptomycin directly into the brain tissues and membranes in tubercular meningitis; the curative effect could also be achieved by introducing streptomycin into the bloodstream by intramuscular injections (as it is done today). Physiologists were reproached for a lack of objectivity and competence in assessing the efficacy of their method in the treatment of other diseases.

And another thing: Stern used her personal contacts to obtain streptomycin in the United States. Believing that difficulties were intentionally put in her way by bureaucrats in the government, she devised ways of bypassing them. In resorting to such measures she was guided, first and foremost, by fanatical faith in the miraculous and universal nature of her cure and also, undoubtedly, by ambition. That was part of her makeup. Stern's brother, who lived in the United States, bought the antibiotic with his own money and, seemingly in circumvention of the law—at any rate he was eventually forced to leave the States a ruined man—mailed it to her. So for a while, Stern had the monopoly on all streptomycin in the Soviet Union and herself doled it out to medical establishments for the treatment of tubercular meningitis, on the condition that it would be conducted according to her method. At one time, Stalin's daughter Svetlana Alliluyeva-Stalin approached her to request some streptomycin for a child of close friends. Stern flatly refused, saying that she received streptomycin not for treating tuberculosis in general but strictly for purposes of research.

Gradually, dark clouds began to gather over Stern's head, although of course she was not alone. There were various symptoms and signals. One was the information passed on to her in confidence that Malenkov and Shcherbakov, close associates of Stalin, were hostile and spoke ill of her. I personally heard the same from Yakov Etinger (subsequently a victim of the Doctors' Plot). Etinger was then attending Shcherbakov, who had just suffered a severe heart attack and died soon afterward. After one of his visits, Shcherbakov invited Etinger to stay for tea. There both Shcherbakov and Malenkov, who was also present, denigrated Stern and her method. One of them, according to Etinger, said: "I am sure that Stern's method has cured no one, and we have been too hasty in making her an academician." Of course this chat had no direct consequences on Stern's fate, which, like that of Etinger himself, was shaped by other circumstances. This is merely an example of the thickening atmosphere that culminated in her arrest.

The arrest was preceded by a number of actions aimed at discrediting her as a scientist. But it would be naive to suggest that her faults as a scientist, real or imaginary, played the decisive role in her destruction. At that time, scientists of stature and unquestionable integrity were demolished before the eyes of one and all ("turned into shit," according to Nikolai Vavilov), while patent ignoramuses were lauded as geniuses and their ravings declared to be the latest word in science. There were any number of ignoramuses and frauds of lesser scope active in the world of Soviet science, and all of them prospered under the benevolent eye of the Stalinist powers.

A certain part in Stern's arrest was probably played by the following circumstance. During World War II, a great contribution to the war effort was made by various public organizations, which rallied the country against a formidable enemy. One such organization was the Jewish Anti-Fascist Committee, which included such outstanding Soviet Jews as the writers Bergelsohn, Perets-Markish, Kvitko, and Fefer, the actors Mikhoels and Zuskin, the head physician of Botkin Hospital Shchimeliovich, the politician Lozovsky, the scientists Nusinov and Frumkin, and others. Stern also joined this committee. In general, she was an exotic bird who had, by mishap, flown into Stalin's empire. She retained her "western" appearance and mannerisms; she did not think it necessary to curb her tongue, and, to top it all, she was Jewish and a member of the Jewish Anti-Fascist Committee. Not that she was particularly conscious of her nationality. She had grown up and been educated in an atmosphere of western internationalism, of religious freethinking. All manifestations of Jewish nationalism were alien to her and even repelled her. She joined the Anti-Fascist Committee for reasons that had nothing to do with a desire to be among "her own."

Professional or moral discrediting of a scientist was not an original device in the arsenal of the security bodies. Remember the episode with Dr. Pletnyov that preceded his arrest and trial in 1938 (publicly accused of sexually assaulting a patient). And the same sort of thing happened with such figures as Bukharin, Rykov, Yagoda, Rosenholtz, Levin, and others.

For Lina Stern, who was then nearly seventy, another method of aspersion was chosen (although sexual allegations were actually made by her investigator). The campaign began with the publication of an article written by a certain Bernstein, head of the department of biochemistry at the Medical Institute in Ivanovo. The article appeared in the summer of 1947 in *Meditsinsky rabotnik*. At that time, this medical newspaper propagandized all brands of scientific obscurantism, with nauseating benightedness, and was the mouthpiece of Black-Hundred-minded slanderers. In his article Bernstein disparaged the research conducted by Stern and her institute in the hematoencephalic barrier. This was more than a hit: it was the first of a deluge of arrows. It could have been written on Bernstein's own initiative, in anticipation of approval from above, or there could have been a more powerful mastermind behind him. At any rate, the arrow hit the political target and was followed in mid-1948 by Medgiz's publication of a booklet by the same Bernstein, under the racy title *Against Simplification and Simplifiers*. This was brought out urgently, ahead of all kinds of books that were really needed and had been awaiting publication for years. From the day his article appeared in *Meditsinsky rabotnik*, Bernstein led the campaign of vilification against Lina Stern. A Jew, he was most suitable for the role, thereby absolving her hounders of charges of antisemitism. His role was for all the world as low as that of the woman who accused Pletnyov of attacking a patient or of Lydia Timashuk in the Doctors' Plot, and undoubtedly it carried a reward. While his booklet was being prepared for publication and for some time afterward, Bernstein was the hero of the day. He was issued a permanent pass to the Central Committee; he could call at any time on Minister of Health Smirnov, to report on developments and receive instructions; and when he entered (also without being announced) the office of Nikolai Anichkov, president of the Academy of Medical Sciences, the venerable academician jumped up from his chair to greet the "honored guest," hand outstretched.

The booklet that denounced Stern's teachings ("pseudo-teachings") came out in the summer of 1948. And even before, in May 1948, Stern was suddenly summoned by the president of the Academy of Sciences, Sergei Vavilov (Nikolai Vavilov's brother), who informed her that a decision had been taken by the presidium of the academy to move her institute to Leningrad and to appoint Academician Konstantin Bykov its director. Representatives of the new director arrived hot on the heels of that conversation, packed up the equipment, apparatus, and library, and all of it, thrown together helter-skelter, was dispatched forthwith to Leningrad. Even a layman, to say nothing of a scientist engaged in experimentation, can easily understand what happens to apparatus, carefully selected and developed over the years to serve specific scientific purposes, ideas, and plans when they are dismantled and turned over to an establishment that is concerned with very different problems. These apparatus become so much scrap metal—and this is precisely what happened. Thus the transfer of Lina Stern's institute to the jurisdiction of a different academy meant in effect its liquidation, disguised as a reorganization. Reorganizations of this kind were all too common at the time and were a method of dealing with establishments that the Soviet government took exception to, and not only in the field of science. In this way, the Institute of Morphology, whose director was Alexei Abrikosov, was reorganized into an Institute of Pharmacology, with a certain Professor Snyakin, a physiologist, appointed its head. The reason for the reorganization was the label "a nest of Virchowianism" that was slapped on by Olga Lepeshinskaya. Such reorganizations also befell theaters directed by people with distinctive artistic personalities (Meyerhold, Tairov, Koonen), journals, and so on. The procedure was tantamount to, say, the reorganization of a Jewish into a gypsy theater, or vice versa.

Whatever euphemism was used to disguise the liquidation of Stern's institute, the fact remained that it ceased to exist. Its staff was disbanded and forced to undertake an almost hopeless search for jobs elsewhere. Hopeless, because many of them bore a double brand—being Jewish and having collaborated with Lina Stern, who was by now completely discredited. Stern herself was left with a staff of four people, including a personal secretary. It was perfectly clear that her downfall was due not so much to her scientific "mistakes" as to the negative and even hostile attitude toward her in the higher echelons.

One of the last, and perhaps the loudest, chords in the prelude to Stern's arrest was a two-day session of the Moscow Society of Physiologists, Biochemists, and Pharmacologists especially devoted to the scientific activities of Academician Lina Stern. It might seem that there was little point in discussing the research done at her institute after it had been dissolved and the research abandoned. The reverse order of events would seem more logical. But apparently the society was guided not by considerations of logic but rather had to carry out an order. This discussion, the outcome of which was preordained, was obviously seen as a form of justification for the measures that had already been taken, as a "democratic formalization" of prior decisions.

There was no need for subtlety and finesse—the cruder the charges, the clearer and more spectacular. The discussion was undoubtedly inspired from above, for nobody would take the responsibility for organizing what amounted to a civil trial of a member of the academy and party member without approval—or some command—from above.

The show was staged according to a script elaborated, it must be presumed, by the MGB and directed from behind the scenes. The official director was Ivan Razenkov, chairman of the Society of Physiologists and member of the Academy of Medical Sciences, who was a distinguished scientist and a decent man, and who had been on good enough terms with Stern. His was indeed a formidable task, and he performed it with the resignation of one who is well aware that his task is unsavory.

I used the word "show" quite deliberately. It was actually a spectacle staged at Moscow University in the anatomy department's auditorium on Mokhovaya Street. The auditorium, which could seat six thousand, was packed. People were sitting on the steps in the aisles, crowding in the doors and outside them in the hallway. The larger share of the audience consisted of students who had come to watch the spectacle, anticipating either a fascinating massacre or a no less fascinating dogfight between well-known scientists. Unusually enough for that time, the sympathies of the audience were with the victim. Not that the young people could form their own judgment of the merits of Stern's research—no, they were guided by an extremely simple consideration: if these people were being persecuted and vilified, then they must be in the right and worthy of support. So the audience rewarded Stern's defenders with stormy applause and booed her attackers. Characteristic of the moral fiber of the young people was also the fact that two graduate students in the department of physiology of the Second Medical Institute (I remember the name of one of them, Latash) refused point-blank to repudiate their scientific supervisor Stern or to cast aspersions upon her. For this stand, they were threatened with expulsion from the YCL and from the institute—a threat that was promptly made good.

The word "show" is also justified in terms of the tendentious casting of parts. There were the grandiloquent accusers—Bernstein (who obviously regarded himself as first fiddle) accompanied by Asratian, Belenky, Negovsky, and Ognev. The speech by Ippolit Davidovsky was more academic in character. Generally, his participation in the show was something of a surprise, since his field of research was very far removed from Stern's. A part in this macabre business had probably been forced on him as a member of the presidium of the Academy of Medical Sciences. He did criticize Stern's work, but unexpectedly concluded his speech with the admission that she had been "doing important research." He undercut it, however, by insufficiently substantiating his conclusions and by taking an uncritical attitude toward the practical methods of treatment she recommended.

Unlike the denunciations, the sporadic speeches in defense of Lina Stern were frowned upon by the leaders of the discussion, who had obviously been instructed to discourage them. At any rate, when I informed the chairman Ivan Razenkov that I would like to take the floor, he tried to talk me out of it, arguing that I had not worked with Stern for many years. To this day, I do not know whether he was motivated by the desire to protect me from possible repercussions or by less altruistic considerations. Nonetheless, I did not heed his advice, even though I had not been on speaking terms with Stern for a long time. But I considered it my duty to raise my voice in her defense, for I regarded the things being done to Stern not merely as her personal tragedy but as a broader social injustice.

For a number of reasons, the discussion did not end in the climax envisaged by the plotters: there was no damning resolution. The board of the society was unable to scrape together the quorum necessary for the adoption of such a resolution. Most members of the board did everything possible to avoid committing themselves.

The logical climax of the meeting came one night in January 1949. At about one in the morning, three "avenging angels" descended on Lina Stern's apartment on Starokonyushenye Lane, where she lived with her elderly housekeeper Katya (from whom we later learned about these events). The two male and one female visitors informed Stern that Beria was inviting her for a chat. Lina Stern was so naive as to believe that it was really a matter of business and said that surely it could wait till morning, particularly since she had just gone to bed. But the messengers insisted that Lavrenty Pavlovich was expecting her now and it was not polite to keep him waiting. Stern then began dressing with the help of Katya and the female agent, who, to Lina's surprise, made a point of carefully examining every item of clothing before letting her put it on. The woman even accompanied her to the bathroom before they left the apartment. Stern was taken away, and there ended the discussion of the scientific achievements of the world's first woman member of two academies. Since she had no close kin entitled to inquire about her or to bring her parcels this was the last we heard of her.

A few hours before that nocturnal visit, Stern had received a telegram from her brother in Vienna, where he was living in poverty after being booted out of the United States. It read as follows: "Alarmed by absence of letters, things being what they are." This "coded" message, as he believed, expressed his prophetic presentiment about the fate of his beloved sister. The telegram naturally was confiscated by the visitors.

Four years passed—the four concluding years of Stalin's dictatorship. Then, at the end of 1952, we received news about Lina Stern in the form of a letter from Jambul (Central Asia). In this letter, she informed her former associates of her whereabouts and asked some one of them to visit her in Jambul. We were all in a quandary. Obviously this was, on the one hand, a plea for assistance from a helpless old woman, who had never been able to orient herself properly even in everyday situations at home. On the other hand, it was a manifestation of Stern's characteristic egocentrism, her inability to take into account the realities of life and people's circumstances. Moreover, it was not someone really close to her she was appealing to, but to her former research associates. It was as if the four years that had passed had changed nothing either in their relationships or in the opportunities available to them in given new situations. In the end, after some cautious consultations (remember it was 1952), Stern's devoted personal secretary Olga Skvortsova ventured to make the trip to Jambul, despite the possible dire consequences and the cost involved.

Lina Stern returned to Moscow in June 1953. She spent the first few days in Moscow at our place, and my wife (her long-time student and associate) and I did our best to make her comfortable. We learned what happened after that terrible night in 1949. She told us her story as disjointed recollections. Several years later, she used to say with alarm that she remembered nothing about this period—it was as if those four awful years had never been. This gap in her memory, I suspect, was the defense mechanism of "motivated forgetting," according to Freud, against a background of progressive arteriosclerosis of the brain. During those early days back in Moscow, Stern was extremely depressed, like a person emerging from a state of psychological shock. From her incoherent snatches of reminiscences, we gathered that she had been arrested for belonging to the Jewish Anti-Fascist Committee. She could not recall what concrete misdeeds she was accused of, and she had never understood what was criminal about that organization. This is not at all surprising. I know from my own experience that absurd accusations have the quality of dementia, and a normal mind finds it difficult to recount such ravings. Moreover, Stern had only a very vague idea of the political nuances of the time, and she might easily have become dazed by the events, especially in conditions where reality was interwoven with fantasy. As she told us, the only admission she made to the investigators was that she had never taken much interest in the committee's affairs, did not concern herself with its activities, and was not properly "vigilant," though as a communist she probably should have been. She knew nothing about the so-called criminal designs of the committee. The only event implanted clearly in her memory was what she regarded as a trial. All the accused, that is, the entire Jewish Anti-Fascist Committee, were there. Most probably, it was not a trial at all but a confrontation of the "criminal group," with cross-examination and cross-checking of their testimonies. At that time, no trial in the usual sense of the word was ever held in such cases. The sentences were passed by a troika, a tribunal consisting of three people, in the absence of the accused and were then made known to each of the accused individually. From what Stern was able to say, that particular trial did not conclude with the passing of sentences.

She told us she had been particularly shocked by the appearance of Lozovsky and Shchimeliovich. They looked terribly ill, and a nurse was on duty beside Shchimeliovich all the time, syringe in hand. He was a broken man. Lozovsky, on the other hand, displayed great courage and retracted all the testimony he had given during the investigation. When the chairman would say, after looking into his file, "But you said something very different during the investigation," Lozovsky retorted, "Surely you know how such testimony is obtained." In particular he said: "I cannot look Dr. Stern in the face after what I said about her at the investigation, and I beg her forgiveness." Apparently, Fefer was the most consistent informer. Lozovsky referred to him as "witness for the prosecution Fefer." Fefer affirmed that Stern had once said with annoyance, "What is a home country?

My home country is Riga." Stern did not deny the words, but said that the investigation was taking them out of context. I must note in this connection that Lina Stern celebrated her birthday twice a year— on August 26, the day she was born, and on March 31, the day of her arrival in the Soviet Union. And she prized the second birthday much higher, saying that the first one was not of her own doing. She always had a party on March 31, considering it her real birthday.

Stern particularly remembered one interrogation session. "You old cunt," said the investigator. "We know what you went abroad every year for. To fuck around right and left." To this she replied, trying to turn the filth into a joke: "It is said of women who behave in a certain way that, before they are forty, they are paid, and after forty they pay themselves. I am far past forty, so if I ever behaved as you suggest, no amount of money would have sufficed to pay for it." The foul-mouthed investigator burst into a paroxysm of obscenities, which were for the most part unintelligible to Lina (remember that she did not have a very good command of Russian and had certainly never heard such obscene language). Since the word "mother" occurred often in this torrent of filth, she asked, "Why do you keep going on about my mother? She's long dead and never had anything to do with the Anti-Fascist Committee." The investigator continued swearing. Then she said, "I have an idea you are abusing my mother, but could you at least explain to me the expression you keep using? I have an idea it is not decent." Foul language was, by the way, one of the accepted investigatory methods, the purpose of which was to impress on the accused that they were not human beings but mere "dog shit." Vasily Parin told me that when Nikolai Vavilov was in the Saratov Prison, he introduced himself to every new cellmate thus: "Vavilov, formerly academician, now dog shit."

Apart from the interrogation sessions, with their abuse and humiliation, the stupefying days at Lubyanka Prison must have been a terrible physical and moral strain on an old woman, who, even when she was free, had been able to cope with the problems of everyday life only with the aid of her friends and housekeeper. It was almost more than she could do to scrub the floor of the cell, which she shared with three other women for a while, to clean up, and to take out the slop pail when her turn came. In the course of her long stay in Lubyanka, the venerable academician was much berated and ridiculed by her cellmates for untidiness.

The most horrible episode Stern recalled was her transfer to Lefortovo Prison, where she was held for twenty days. She characterized that special-regime prison as hell. Apparently she was placed in a punishment cell, since she had to remain standing the whole day long, though, from my own experience, I can say that the sitting position in a solitary cell of that prison was not that much more comfortable. Stern told us that in Lefortovo she had hallucinations and was quite sure that she was going mad. After that, she was taken back to the comparative comfort of Lubyanka. In the final period of her stay there, her life was somewhat better. She was given paper and pen and allowed to continue her scientific writing. She was allowed to take her notes with her to Jambul, and she brought them back to Moscow—a thick packet of handwritten pages devoted to her favorite subject, the hematoencephalic barrier. I had a look at those notes and was convinced they were of no scientific value whatsoever.

We now know that the case of the Jewish Anti-Fascist Committee ended in the execution of all its members; they were shot on August 12, 1952. The only one spared was Lina Stern. It is hard to guess the reason for this leniency; undoubtedly it had nothing to do with considerations of mercy. She was sentenced to a term of exile (five years) in Central Asia, without confiscation of property. She was even offered a choice of locality. She named Alma-Ata, the capital of Kazakhstan, where she had lived during the war, but her request was rejected—capital cities were off limits. So she landed in Jambul. The money and jewelry taken from her during arrest were returned to her, and she was also allowed to use the money in her bank account.

Still, being an extremely impractical woman, she felt lost in a strange town. Some shady characters latched on to her and, taking advantage of her trustfulness, stole all her jewelry, of which she had quite a lot. Thus the prophecies of her friends in Geneva when she was leaving for the Soviet Union all came true, except that she was exiled not to Siberia but to Central Asia.

After her return to Moscow, Lina Stern got back her two rooms in the communal apartment house on Starokonyushenye Lane, which had been sealed up during the intervening years. Clouds of moths swarmed out of the wardrobes when we opened the doors. She also got back her dacha, and her everyday life gradually returned to normal. She had never been expelled from the Academy of Sciences, and when the salary that had accumulated during her absence (500 rubles a month for an academician) was paid to her, she became rich overnight.

The restoration of her political status, however, proceeded at a much slower place. She had only been amnestied in 1953 and was not reinstated in the party until rehabilitation was formally substituted for the amnesty. But at last this hurdle was overcome too. A special decision of the academy's presidium permitted her to set up a laboratory to continue her research, and the necessary assistance was given to her. The laboratory was organized, and her old staff members came back. They did fruitful research and earned a reputation as a major scientific center, elaborating upon the problem of barrier mechanisms in the human body. Several national conferences, attended by a large number of specialists, were held to discuss the problem. Lina Stern died in the spring of 1968, just a few months short of her ninetieth birthday. In the fall of 1978, a special conference was convened to mark the centenary of the birth of Academician Lina Stern, a remarkable individual and scientist whose memory is kept by the few who remain of her students, colleagues, and friends.

OLGA LEPESHINSKAYA
The Vital Substance and Its Inglorious Demise

THE NAME OF Olga Borisovna Lepeshinskaya was known to every literate Soviet person in the middle of the twentieth century. She was glorified by poets, and plays were written about her by not-too-scrupulous playwrights and performed in numerous theaters. In school and university textbooks, she was described as the author of the greatest discovery in biology, and the essence of the discovery became a compulsory part of courses in Darwinism. Her name, elevated by Stalin to the pinnacle of scientific glory, became, at the same time, a symbol of the mire into which Soviet science had sunk.

The heroine herself, Olga Lepeshinskaya, was a smallish old woman who walked with a limp and used a cane. Her tiny sharp-nosed face, deeply wrinkled, was adorned by spectacles through which she peered myopically at the world, sometimes good-naturedly and occasionally with anger; on the whole she was a mild enough person. Even at the zenith of her fame, the woman appeared somewhat unkempt. Her clothes were old-fashioned and cheap; on her cardigan was invariably pinned a brass brooch of the steamboat *Komsomol*, which had been torpedoed by the Francoists during the civil war in Spain. I once said to Lepeshinskaya that her bosom did not offer the hapless boat the quiet haven it deserved. She did not resent jokes at her expense—I must say that for her.

Olga Lepeshinskaya's biography is indeed quite remarkable and must be viewed on two planes, one quite independent of the other. The same applies to her character. One plane is her life as a veteran communist, a person reared on the principles of Bolshevism. Lep-

254

eshinskaya, and particularly her husband Panteleimon Lepeshinsky, had been friends and associates of Lenin and his wife Nadezhda Krupskaya (they had all been banished to the same region of Siberia between 1897 and 1900), and their lives intertwined with Lenin's on occasion. Lepeshinskaya often spoke at meetings about Lenin and wrote reminiscences of him, which supplemented our knowledge of the leader of the Russian revolution as a man.

Lepeshinskaya had many likeable qualities, primarily democratism, for she treated all people alike regardless of social standing. She was forthright and outspoken, with complete disregard for the rank of her opponent, and she had an extreme distaste for every manifestation of antisemitism. In fact, the most crushing thing she could say of a person was, "he's a Judophobe" (she used this prerevolutionary term for antisemitism). She was amiable and good-natured, and she brought up several orphans (some six or eight, I believe) who were her adopted grandchildren and to whom she gave an education and a start in life. But she put her Bolshevik staunchness to very bad use when she launched the campaign for her pseudo-scientific concepts. Supported by the all-powerful Lysenko, she turned her militancy against the true interests of science and against its finest representatives.

The entire family of Lepeshinskaya, her daughter Olga, her son-in-law Vladimir Kryukov, and even her adopted granddaughter Svetlana, who was then about twelve, were members of her research team. The only person who kept away from this family team was her husband Panteleimon, who died before the family hit the headlines. Moreover, he never concealed his skeptical, even ironic, attitude to the scientific dabblings of his spouse. Once I met the couple on a commuter train to the countryside, and the whole trip long Olga spouted her scientific theories at me. Panteleimon listened apathetically; no emotion could be detected on the kind, wise face of this intellectual with the characteristic gray goatee. But at one point he said to me in his mild voice: "Don't you listen to her, she's totally ignorant about science, and everything she's been saying is a lot of rubbish." Olga did not even attempt to refute this appraisal—apparently she had heard her husband express it before. Nor did her husband's words put a stop to her scientific outpourings. So she kept on jabbering away, and her husband watched the passing scenery through the window with complete detachment.

Her daughter and son-in-law were members of the Cytological

Laboratory at the Institute of Morphology which was headed by Lepeshinskaya. They were scientific zeroes, mere satellites of their volcanic mother. I am not even sure they both had university degrees—perhaps only Kryukov did (they were about forty at the time I am describing). As for the daughter, one only had to talk to her for a few minutes to know that she was altogether ignorant in the scientific sphere in which she was supposed to be doing research.

Lepeshinskaya's laboratory was located in the Government Building by the Stone Bridge, where the Lepeshinskys, both veteran party members, were allotted two apartments—one as living quarters and the other to be used as a laboratory. So Lepeshinskaya and her family team could work practically without leaving their kitchen. Naturally such a laboratory lacked all the complicated equipment and apparatus necessary for doing research at the cellular level, and particularly for coping with the mammoth tasks Lepeshinskaya set herself. Nor did she feel any need for complicated equipment, for she was quite sure she could solve biology's most fundamental problems with the most primitive of methods.

Once, at Lepeshinskaya's insistent invitation, I visited her laboratory. I had known her for many years and was, in fact, a friend of hers, but this particular visit was made in my official capacity as deputy director for research of the Institute of Morphology. The reception was of course cordial, and they had obviously taken great pains to impress me favorably. But I could see that it was all window-dressing. There was feverish activity going on in the laboratory, undoubtedly intended to disprove the many rumors about the monumental sloth prevailing there. I was shown the equipment, pride of place belonging to an electric drying cupboard imported from England (at that time foreign-made equipment was accessible only to the chosen few). Two young laboratory assistants in clean (as yet unlaundered) overalls were pounding something in china mortars. When I asked Lepeshinskaya's daughter what it was they were pounding, she said it was beetroot seeds. The purpose was to obtain confirmation of the theory that not only those sections of a plant ovule which included the embryo could germinate, but any segment could do so, inasmuch as all contained the "vital substance." Then she acquainted me with her own current line of research: "We take dirt from under Mama's nails and study it for the vital substance." I took this to be a joke but then gathered that such nonsense was actually regarded as a serious

256

experiment to prove that living organisms could be engendered from dead matter. It became just another in a series of pseudo-scientific "discoveries" launched into the scientific world.

One such discovery was made by Boshian, who claimed that he had established the laws governing the transformation of viruses into microscopically visible bacterial forms, as well as their transformation into a crystalline form capable of further vegetation. It was proved soon enough that all his discoveries were nothing but the fruit of profound ignorance and neglect of all the elementary rules of bacteriology, rules known even to schoolchildren. But to begin with, until proven otherwise, Boshian's discovery was lauded as a revolution in microbiology on a par with similar revolutions wrought by Lysenko and Lepeshinskaya. A major administrator of the health ministry even went so far as to announce at a serious scientific gathering, brandishing Boshian's little booklet: "The old microbiology is dead. Here is the new microbiology for you!" Were we to understand that the microbiology of Pasteur, Koch, Ehrlich, and other giants had been replaced by Boshian's? This particular scientific charlatan was unlucky in that he did not secure the support of Lysenko and Lepeshinskaya. The latter even accused him of plagiarism of her own work, speaking of Boshian with the scorn generally reserved for a petty thief. That particular luminary ended his career by being stripped of all his academic ranks and degrees.

To return to my visit to Lepeshinskaya's laboratory, I left with the impression that I had been looking into the pots of a medieval alchemist, only to learn some time later that I had been granted the honor of being admitted to Olympus. What was the essence of Lepeshinskaya's discovery? Here I must introduce the reader to some elementary principles of biology and medicine.

Until the discovery of the cellular structure of organisms, there existed the mystical concept of *blastema*, which was supposed to contain all the vital properties and of which all tissues of any living organism, however complex, were formed. As microscopic technology was perfected, Schleiden discovered cells in plants (1836), and Schwann, in animals (1838). The cell was accepted as the elementary unit of a living organism. This was one of the great discoveries of the nineteenth century. Subsequently, the German scientist Remak formulated the law of neoplasia and growth of tissues, according to which every cell is engendered by a mother cell by division; amorphous blastema could not be the origin of this complicated structure. Nonformalized intracellular matter can be considered a derivative of cell function, although no one denies the importance of its role in physiology and pathology.

The great German scientist Rudolf Virchow applied the cellular principle to the analysis of disease. In his book *Cellular Pathology* (1858) he formulated his views as an integrated theory. The publication of this book was a milestone in the history of medicine, dividing it into two periods: pre-Virchowian and Virchowian. "All pathology is pathology of the cell," Virchow declared. "The cell is the cornerstone in the edifice of scientific medicine." His cellular theory of the origin of disease replaced the humoral theory, which dated back to Hippocrates. The older theory held that the development of a disease was the result of a change in the organism's "juices." Even the most consistent proponent of the humoral theory, Karl Rokitansky, admitted that Virchow's cellular theory was far superior, inasmuch as it provided an actual substrate for disease, the cell, instead of the vague notion of *dyscrasias* (changes in the juices). Cellular theory represented a complex system of views that were criticized even in Virchow's lifetime by Russian scientists, among others, in particular by Ivan Sechenov. What is important is that Virchow's theory completely supports and develops the data obtained by Remak concerning the proliferation of old cells into new ones, which was formulated by Virchow as: "Omnis cellula e cellulae" (each cell from a cell). This formula was later complemented by the words "ejusdem generis" (of the same genus). The addition stipulated that the newly formed cells had the generic properties of the parent cell, determined by the genetic code contained in the chromosome apparatus of the cell's nucleus.

Virchow's cellular pathology had a profound effect on medicine and biology and gave a powerful impetus to their development. This impetus has not exhausted itself to this day, in particular, as regards the laws of the cellular structure of organisms, which Virchow applied to pathology and medicine. Now Olga Lepeshinskaya claimed to have disproved the foundations of cellular theory. According to her, the basic properties of an organism were contained not in the cell but in some amorphous "vital substance." This substance was the bearer of all vital processes and it formed cells, with all their complex subcellular structures. Lepeshinskaya did not bother to ascertain the nature of this vital substance—it was only a vague, semimystical concept.

In Lepeshinskaya's opinion, her studies dealt a crushing blow to the greatest discovery of the nineteenth century, to cellular theory in general and to Virchow's formula "each cell from a cell" in particular. She dismissed all biologists who did not agree with her as stubborn and ignorant Virchowians. This label, which had denigrating political as well as scientific connotations, was not her own invention. It was concocted by a band of incompetents who styled themselves authors of a new trend in pathology. The label was similar in implications to Weismanist, Mendelist, and Morganist, which Lysenko and his cohorts slapped onto geneticists. Lepeshinskaya's vital-substance theory dragged the science of biology back to the times of blastema.

Throughout the history of science, researchers have reverted to old, seemingly outdated theories. But such reversions occurred as a new coil on the spiral of scientific advancement and represented a higher stage of progress. The adage that the new is the well-forgotten old is often justified. But this advancement along a spiral is based on continuously perfected equipment, given technological progress in general. Lepeshinskaya's work did not meet this primary requirement. Her methods were so primitive and nonprofessional that all the proofs she could offer in support of her theory tumbled down at the first critical glance.

Her main object of study was egg yolk, which contains no cells and is simply a nutrient medium for the chicken embryo. But it was in egg yolk that Lepeshinskaya discovered formation of cells out of the vital substance. When I examined her histological specimens, I became convinced that her conclusion was reached only through crude defects in histological technique. Nevertheless, although several specialists gave a similar negative assessment of her proofs, she wrote a book in which she summed up her research and which, as she told me, she intended to dedicate to Stalin. Stalin declined the honor but regarded the book itself with favor, lending his support to its ideas. This determined the subsequent course of events.

The attitude of the academic community to Lepeshinskaya's discovery was initially unambiguous. A group of prominent histologists and biologists from Leningrad, which included such distinguished scientists as Dmitry Nasonov, Vasily Alexandrov, Nikolai Khlopin, and

Dmitry Knorre, twelve persons in all, published a letter in *Meditsinsky rabotnik* in which they subjected Lepeshinskaya's work to annihilating criticism. Her conclusions were described as the product of crass ignorance and methodological ineptness. The editors of the newspaper, impressed by the eminence of the authors, published the letter since the attitude of the party and government leadership to Lepeshinskaya's work had not been officially declared. So retribution against the writers of the letter, who were fighting for the purity of science, was delayed until Lepeshinskaya was crowned queen of biology.

Lepeshinskaya's discoveries were not confined to the vital substance. She also gave humanity the gift of her soda baths, which, she claimed, returned youth to the old and helped the young remain young. She spoke of this panacea at a sitting of the Academic Council of the Institute of Morphology in 1948 or 1949, which was chaired by Alexei Abrikosov. The audience—the most distinguished morphologists of Moscow—was literally staggered by Lepeshinskaya's announcement. She made no attempt to substantiate the effect of soda baths (she just mumbled some generalities about the vital substance) but instead described the wonderful results obtained at the Barvikha Sanatorium, an upper-echelon establishment for party leaders, old Bolsheviks, major scientists, writers, and actors. Lepeshinskaya spoke at length about the favorable comments these elitarians had made about the effect of soda baths. One felt ashamed—both for the speaker and for the audience forced to listen to these imbecilities. After Lepeshinskaya finished, an oppressive silence hung over all. Abrikosov, looking around the audience imploringly, proposed that we ask questions. Finally I decided to relieve the tension by a naughty question, which was quite in keeping with my usual ironic attitude to Olga: "Will mineral water work just as well?" Lepeshinskaya, oblivious of the sarcasm, gave me a matter-of-fact answer to the effect that soda could not be replaced by mineral water.

Her idea about soda baths was widely publicized, and baking soda disappeared from the shops. This was yet another manifestation of the mass hysteria of the times. Even critically minded people half-believed the propaganda and decided to make an attempt at rejuvenation. Soon, however, the hysteria died down and soda reappeared. Nothing but jokes remained to remind us of yesterday's miracle-working panacea.

The soda-bath paper caused a rift between Lepeshinskaya and the party organization at the Institute of Morphology. The party secretary Dora Komissaruk launched an attack on Lepeshinskaya over the vapidity of her research, the nepotism of her home laboratory, and the absence of even elementary discipline. I didn't have such strong feelings, reflecting that Lepeshinskaya had been a fine revolutionary and that science was not a profession but a hobby for her—a harmless folly that could be overlooked since age itself (she was then nearly eighty) would soon put an end to it. So my attitude was one of humorous indulgence, which was most clearly expressed in the proposal I made to Lepeshinskaya after her "coronation." As I sat chatting with some of my colleagues in the blue drawing room of the Scientists' Club, Olga Lepeshinskaya, with her walking cane, entered the room, her head held arrogantly high as always. I said, "Olga, may I join the ranks of your admirers? Do consent to be my wife, and we shall make children of the vital substance." This joke, I later learned, was repeated with delight throughout the academic community. I felt sure that no self-respecting scientist would debate her findings, since there were no findings to debate. Events proved me wrong, however. It turned out that Lepeshinskaya did not regard her pseudo-scientific activities as a hobby at all, for the old woman was consumed by a mammoth ambition and aspired to make no less than a revolution in the science of biology.

As the result of her conflict with the party organization, Lepeshinskaya was forced to leave the Institute of Morphology, and she nursed a grudge about this to the end of her days. Her entire laboratory was transferred to the Institute of Experimental Biology of the Academy of Medical Sciences, whose director Ivan Maisky, and his deputy Nikolai Zhukov-Verezhnikov, undoubtedly regarded Lepeshinskaya as a means of furthering their own careers. With their help (and support from above), Lepeshinskaya was able to see her dream come true. The revolution in biology was sponsored by Lysenko and decreed by the Soviet leadership.

By order of the Central Committee, a special closed-door conference was held to discuss Lepeshinskaya's work. The participants were hand-picked from among biologists who could be induced to cooperate. In preparation for the conference, pains were taken to support her conclusions with adequate experimental evidence. Since Lepeshinskaya's own specimens, which she regarded as conclusive, were not fit to be demonstrated, Professor Grigory Khrushchev was asked to provide professional histological specimens that would be suitable for a superficial examination through a microscope. And so, on May 22–24, 1950, a most disgraceful show was staged at the department of biology of the Soviet Academy of Sciences, titled "Conference on the Problem of the Vital Substance and the Development of Cells." It was chaired by Academician Alexander Oparin, head of the academy's department of biology. His speech was the overture, so to speak, to a comedy that was performed by a chosen cast of twenty-seven scientists to an audience of over a hundred specially invited persons. The names of these performers were immortalized in the short-hand minutes of the proceedings (published by the Academy of Sciences in 1950 and on which I have based this account). Many participants realized that a shameful role was being foisted upon them. In later years, they tried their best to wash themselves clean of the dirt, but the fact remains that there was not one Giordano Bruno among them. That is, there might have been Brunos and Galileos among Soviet biologists, but they were not admitted: participants were, after all, carefully selected for maximal obedience.

After Oparin's overture came the family trio, which consisted of Olga Lepeshinskaya, her daughter Olga, and her son-in-law Vladimir Kryukov. There was also somebody named Sorokin, a staff member from Lepeshinskaya's laboratory who had a veterinarian's diploma and was obviously a psychopath. He read a miserable little paper, which had nothing to do with the vital substance and which he had composed while taking a graduate course in Lina Stern's Institute of Physiology. He must have been chosen to speak at the conference only on the strength of his devotion to Lepeshinskaya: better a quartet than a trio. I shall not discuss their papers: any sober scientific look would have annihilated them. The paper by the elder Lepeshinskaya was packed with abuse of Virchowians, philosophical and political demagogy, and endless references to Marxist-Leninist teachings, particularly Stalin's works. The concluding passage must be quoted verbatim, since it contains the essence of the paper and would have done very well in its stead: "In conclusion, I want to express my heartfelt gratitude to our great teacher and friend, that scholar of incomparable genius, the leader of advanced science, our dear Comrade Stalin. His teaching, his every pronouncement on the problems of science, was for me an inspiration and provided immense support in my long-standing and bitter struggle against the monopolists in science—idealists of all brands and hues. Long live our great Stalin, the great leader of the world proletariat and all progressive mankind!"

At that time, many reports and speeches ended on this note. It was a kind of demagogic shield used by incompetents to protect themselves from scientific criticism, and it always evoked thunderous applause. Just try criticizing something after such an explosion of approval! I knew one professor who was rebuked for the poor delivery of his lectures and their inadequate scientific content in general. This he indignantly denied, saying that the audience invariably cheered his lectures. And so they did, because he concluded each one with a reference to the genius of Stalin, by whose beneficence the incidence of the disease he was discussing had been greatly lowered. This was a stereotyped device for the times, one that was infallibly effective. It has a literary prototype in Chekhov's story about the police officer's wife who, whenever her husband started scolding her, sat down at the piano and played the hymn "God Save the Tsar." At the first chord, the police officer fell silent, stood at attention, and saluted.

Lepeshinskaya, moreover, had every reason to express her gratitude to Stalin, since she had received his blessing (direct or indirect, through Lysenko); without it her claim to the title of reformer of biology would elicit merely a pitying smile. I must confess that for a long time I regarded her discoveries as ludicrous pretensions that did not merit serious opposition, until the conference and what followed convinced me that the ludicrous claim was a serious threat to science and scientists.

I will not quote from the conference speeches of the twenty-seven troubadours who sang of Lepeshinskaya. Their eulogies differed only in degree of obsequiousness. Almost no one attempted an analysis, even a favorable one, of the actual evidence offered. They were not interested in facts (nor were they competent to assess them). They simply accepted her claim as irrefutably proven. All that remained was to hold forth on the general philosophy of the natural sciences and on the importance of Lepeshinskaya's discovery. Among these eulogists were toadies, frauds, and ignoramuses, for whom this frail old woman was but a powerful springboard to academic and administrative advancement. Their participation in this deplorable show was quite in order and not at all surprising.

Much sadder was the role played by major scientists, supposedly men of integrity, such as the academicians Pavlovsky, Anichkov, Imshenetsky, Speransky, Timakov, Davidovsky, and Severin. Their participation was required to lend the spectacle academic prestige. These people were of course aware of what was going on, since the Central Committee had already received their agreement to support Lepeshinskaya. The only total fool was Trofim Lysenko. Lepeshinskaya's discoveries were cooked up according to the same recipe as Lysenko's: these two giants richly deserved each other. In his speech Lysenko repeated the fundamental tenets of his theory, the worth of which can be judged from this quotation: "Abundant factual material has now been accumulated which testifies that rye can be engendered by wheat—and different grades of wheat too. The same grades of wheat can also produce barley. Rye too can produce wheat. Oats can produce wild oats . . ." How is this bacchanalia of transformations set into motion? Lysenko found the answer in Lepeshinskaya's discovery. "Lepeshinskaya's work," he said, "showing that cells need not be formed from other cells but can also be formed from noncellular matter, helps us construct a theory of species transformation." Lysenko's idea was not simply that a wheat plant cell is transformed into a rye plant cell. According to Lepeshinskaya's theory, he represents the process like this: "In the body of a wheat plant, under the influence of definite growing conditions, grains of rye are formed . . . In the depth of the plant body of the given species, out of a substance that is not cellular in structure [the vital substance], grains of another species are engendered. Of these, subsequently, cells and embryos of another species are formed. This is the contribution of Olga Lepeshinskaya's work to the development of the theory of species formation." As I reread these lines, I remembered the assistants in Lepeshinskaya's laboratory who were pounding beetroot seeds. So that must have been the experimental confirmation of the greatest discovery in biology.

The most restrained speech at the conference was made by Nikolai Anichkov, president of the Academy of Medical Sciences. He did not extol Lepeshinskaya's discoveries but only gave a brief precis, saying that he had seen some of the specimens [prepared by Grigory Khrushchev] but had not had a chance to study them thoroughly. "I was shown structures and transformations," he said, "which really may be regarded as evidence of the engendering of cells from noncellular vital substance. But of course it is desirable that more such data should be accumulated on different objects . . . This is the ultimate condition for accepting new positions in biology. The factual aspect must be represented as fully as possible, so that the new views might be accepted even by those scientists who maintain the opposite stand." Further, he politely gave Lepeshinskaya her due for the persistent struggle she had waged to have her discovery acknowledged and said that favorable conditions must be created for her work.

The other speakers were less scrupulous and declared the experimental specimens offered by Lepeshinskaya to be wholly conclusive. I was particularly surprised by the speech of Ippolit Davidovsky, member of the Academy of Medical Sciences and one of the leaders of Soviet pathology. I shall quote the beginning and end of his address. The beginning: "Olga Lepeshinskaya's book, her paper and demonstration, as well as the speeches of the other participants, left me personally in no doubt that she is on the right path." The end: "In conclusion I feel obliged to give my thanks to Olga Lepeshinskaya on behalf of all Soviet pathologists for her pointed criticism and for the fresh spirit she has infused into science. I am sure this will create new prospects for the development of Soviet pathology." I later heard that Davidovsky said he had received direct orders from "the highest quarters."

Academician Alexei Speransky virtually groveled before Lepeshinskaya for the courage with which she had overcome the resistance of her ideological opponents. His speech consisted of delirious praise and was devoid of all scientific content whatever. Here is an excerpt: "Only an old Bolshevik like Olga Lepeshinskaya would have the strength to surmount the mockery and finally produce such proofs as leave no room for doubt. I personally would have been sorely grieved if—for the sole reason of methodological shortcomings—Lepeshinskaya's cause, the cause of all Soviet science, had been discredited, if our science had become the object of scorn on the part of persons always ready to jeer." The phrase concealed an autobiographical reference. He was taking revenge for the mockery his own discoveries had repeatedly provoked. Not too scrupulous in establishing proofs, and inclined to draw far-reaching conclusions from insufficient data, Speransky measured Lepeshinskaya's work with the same yardstick, cynically asserting that one did not need incontestable proof to create a theory. If there were no such proof, so much the worse for the theory's opponents, not for the theory. In light of such an assertion, how can I be too hard on my graduate student Lydia Ishchenko, who claimed that what was important in a thesis was correct conclusions—and that any fool could collect research materials. But Ishchenko was a sick person, suffering from a severe form of schizophrenia, while here was a mentally healthy academician ending his florid speech with what amounted to a declaration of love: "We must admit our responsibility for the cause of Olga Lepeshinskaya and must do our best to lighten the burden which is lying on the frail shoulders of our darling Olga."

Only two speakers at the conference touched on the quality of the factual material that lay at the basis of Lepeshinskaya's discovery. One was Grigory Khrushchev, director of the academy's Institute of the Morphology of Development, who was soon after elected corresponding member of the academy. He had prepared the histological specimens demonstrated at the conference, so naturally he attested to their authenticity. In conclusion Khrushchev spoke of the need to uproot the survivals of Virchowianism and Weismanism and finished with the usual paean: "Lepeshinskaya's work conclusively demonstrates that, following the precepts of the Leninist-Stalinist teaching on development, it is possible to discover the real laws of the organic world."

Another professor, Mikhail Baron, head of the department of histology of the First Medical Institute, said that the specimens prepared by Khrushchev had persuaded him of the correctness of Lepeshinskaya's inferences. I cannot say what induced him, a major specialist who was extremely exacting in questions of morphological methodology and was himself a past master at it, who had formerly rejected Lepeshinskaya's work out of hand, to change his mind. I suppose he yielded to pressure from above, to which he had always been sensitive; another factor might have been his trust in the work of his colleague, Khrushchev. Subsequently he was cruelly punished for such trustfulness by Lepeshinskaya herself, whose assistant, Sorokin, accused him of scientific plagiarism. The charge was supported by Lepeshinskaya and Davidovsky, with the usual consequences for Baron.

In a word, this was no academically scrupulous forum that approached the experimental materials and the conclusions based on them with strict objectivity, but a carefully staged farce of collective ecstasy for the "great discovery." Unfortunately, there was no child among the participants to exclaim with naive truthfulness that the

266

empress wore no clothes. The doors were locked to keep those naive children out, and there was not one devotee of science in the audience who was prepared to sacrifice a career for its sake. No, there were no would-be martyrs.

The question naturally arises: how were scientists induced to agree to the shameful roles they played at that conference? I imagine that two factors were at work, psychological and sociopolitical. The psychological factor consisted in selecting people who were known to be complaisant to orders from above and were accustomed to executing them unquestioningly. This was the clique of scientists who enjoyed favor with the leadership and prized this favor above all else for the privileges it entailed. Conscious or unconscious fear of losing these privileges was the motive behind many base actions. The psychological factor also manifested itself in another form. Some scientists did not consciously perform such actions but were hypnotized, as it were, and lost their bearings. Indeed, one had to have a most independent and sober mind to keep calm amidst these orgies of triumphant ignorance, to remain true to the criteria of real science while waiting patiently for its time to return.

Forcing scientists to play a base role was but one part of the general system of corruption of knowledge and culture practiced by Stalin's regime—corruption that involved the destruction of the traditional virtues of uprightness, kindness, courage, and honesty, all components, in short, of conscience. It was thanks to this system that the crown of scientific genius was placed on Lepeshinskaya's poor head. The farcical conference unanimously recognized her work as conclusive and revolutionary. She was awarded the Stalin Prize and elected to the Academy of Medical Sciences. Thus the revolution in biological sciences was formalized; thus an act of no longer individual but collective shamelessness was consummated. This triumph of obscurantism occurred in 1950, in the age of the atom, space exploration, and great discoveries (real ones) in biology. The vital substance proved stronger than Reason.

Now all the mechanisms of propaganda were set into motion—prose, poetry, radio, television, the theater. I think only the composers failed to make a contribution. The duty of quoting Lepeshinskaya's teaching at every lecture was imposed upon professors in the medical disciplines, and a strict check was kept to see that they did so.

I was not present at the scientific conference held in the Hall of

Columns of the House of Trade Unions. But I was told by those who attended that Lepeshinskaya was given a standing ovation. I suppose only a small portion of the applause was sincere. The others merely yielded to the herd instinct. All but the most sober were swept off their feet by this stream of adulation. How could one reproach a woman nearing eighty for the fact that the remains of her critical self-appraisal, if she was ever capable of such, had been swept away? She wanted to see the scientific world at her feet, especially that section of it which had refused to acknowledge her achievements. And so the every-ready apparatus/ of power came down heavily on those opponents. The first to suffer were the Leningrad scientists. But Lepeshinskaya did not deny absolution to those who repented of their sins. Professor Knorre, who had been among her most vehement critics, went to see her and, after lingering by the door for a few seconds, rushed to her with open arms, as she herself told me afterward. She embraced him readily, had a short chat, and then saw him on his way with the evangelical injunction: "Go now, and sin no more." She told me about Knorre's visit with great complacency and expressed her secret desire that Nikolai Khlopin, one of her most stubborn opponents, should do penance as well. At this point, my customary ironies toward her failed for the first time, and I retorted harshly that she would never live to see the day. The conversation ended in a violent quarrel, during which I told her in so many words what I thought of her discovery. She countered with screams (this was no longer a meek old lady but an enraged tigress) that a big prize had been promised in the United States to whomever could disprove her theory, while in Czechoslovakia four laboratories had already confirmed it. I replied that even if things were as she said, then people would be making money on her—in America by disproving her and in Czechoslovakia by approving her. This was one of our last meetings (the summer of 1951), and it was witnessed by chance by my neighbor Kaplan, a noted economist. The reverberations of that quarrel reached me in Lefortovo Prison two years later, all the way from the city of Frunze in Central Asia. As for my forecast about Nikolai Khlopin's behavior, I was proved wrong: in the end he had to acknowledge Lepeshinskaya's discovery in order to save his laboratory, but the strain proved too much: he soon fell ill and died.

Another of Lepeshinskaya's major opponents also had to give in to her: Academician Dmitry Nasonov, a proud man and a scientific aristocrat. I had to witness his humiliation twice. The first episode took place soon after Lepeshinskaya's coronation, at a time when he and his assistants came under fire for their heresy. I saw him sitting in the hall of the Academy of Medical Sciences at the desk normally occupied by an employee of the academy, Bella Semyonovna. Semyonovna was absent, and Nasonov was sitting at her desk, reading a novel, and from time to time using the telephone to dial the number of Zhdanov, head of the science section in the Central Committee. Nasonov expected to be received by Zhdanov and relied greatly on his support. As was customary among the top people then, they never simply refused to see a person through their secretaries. The secretary would say that her boss was at a conference, absent, or engaged and ask the person to call again in half an hour. It was not proper to deny an audience to an academician; one had to give some reason, and they all followed the hypocritical bureaucratic procedure. And so Academician Nasonov spent the entire day sitting at Semyonovna's desk, answering her calls with the formula that was very much like the one he was himself being subjected to: "Bella Semyonovna is out right now. I don't know when she'll be back. Please call again in half an hour."

The second case I saw of Nasonov's humiliation occurred at a session of the Academy of Sciences in summer 1951, held at the Scientists' Club in Moscow. He made a "penitent" speech there (by the way, one had first to receive the authorities' permission to repent—an assurance that repentance would be accepted). Immediately afterwards, he dashed into the foyer and, covering his face with his hands, sobbed: "How shameful! How shameful!" I tried to comfort him with the formula Miron Vovsi had coined: "Nothing is shameful nowadays."

And what response did Lepeshinskaya's discovery receive abroad? I was only able to judge from the East German journal *Zentralblatt allgemeine Pathologie und pathologische Anatomie* (during the campaign against "obsequiousness to the west" we had practically no access to foreign journals). This particular issue carried information, without comment, about Lepeshinskaya's discovery and methodology (Grenacher's technique of staining histological specimens with borax carmine). Information about the use of this elementary method, developed in the nineteenth century, to make an epochal-making discovery of the twentieth century was followed by an exclamation mark in brackets. The exclamation mark was the journal's only comment on the discovery.

The restrained skepticism of East German pathologists did not, however, provide a model for the leading party and government bodies in other socialist countries. Following a command from the center, they acknowledged the discoveries of Lysenko and Lepeshinskaya as great achievements upon which scientists in their own countries were to base their research. Characteristic in this respect is the testimony of the eminent Polish physicist Leopold Infeld, a student and associate of Albert Einstein's. For many years Infeld lived and worked in the United States and Canada until, in 1950, at the invitation of the Polish government, he returned to Poland. He writes in his memoirs (published by *Novy mir* in 1965) how puzzled he was, being accustomed to independent scientific work, by the command of the Polish government to take Lysenko and Lepeshinskaya's ideas as guidelines in all his research. Infeld wrote that he was particularly dismayed by the inauguration speech made by the newly appointed first president of the Polish Academy of Sciences, Jan Dembowski. In that speech Dembowski urged Polish scientists to follow the path blazed by Lysenko and Lepeshinskaya—not, mind you, the path blazed by such luminaries of Polish science as Marie Sklodowska-Curie and Marian Smoluchowski. From Infeld's memoirs one gets a clear picture of the government intervention in science that was practiced in all socialist countries in the period of the personality cult.

After her coronation, Lepeshinskaya did not rest on her laurels. She made yet another discovery, into the mysteries of which she initiated me during one of our meetings in the countryside. She had come to the conclusion that television was harmful to the vital substance. She did not say how she established this, but, in her everlasting concern for the welfare of humanity, she informed the powers-that-be of the danger. An alarmed "television director," as she referred to him, came to see her and was deeply impressed. But her warning did not seem to affect television visibly. Apparently in this field, praxis was allowed to lag behind science.

The ideas of Olga Lepeshinskaya, and even of her daughter, were forced on research establishments everywhere. Very active in this respect was the vice-president of the Academy of Medical Sciences, Nikolai Zhukov-Verezhnikov. Adepts of Lepeshinskaya's teaching surfaced in all the research establishments, for this was the surest road to academic success. Careerism was given right' of way, as was duping the gullible.

An example of this duping is provided by the article of a certain

Professor Melkonian, head of the surgery department at the Medical Institute in Yerevan, which was published in 1951 by the journal of the Academy of Sciences *Uspekhi sovremennoi biologii* (Achievements of Modern Biology), edited by Alexander Studitsky, another supporter of Lysenko's and Lepeshinskaya's theories. Melkonian wrote that a jar with echinococcus cysts preserved in formalin had been kept in the modest museum of his department. He had extracted those cysts during an operation on a patient's femur. For many years he had been showing the jar to his students at lectures, and in all that time the cysts did not change in appearance. But once, in preparation for a lecture, he took the jar from the shelf and discovered that the cysts had disappeared; instead of the clear formalin, there was a strange brown liquid with a nasty smell and some bones. At first, he wrote, he decided that somebody had played a practical joke on him, but then it occurred to him that he might be witnessing an experiment staged by Nature itself and that he was duty-bound to examine the matter more deeply. He took the bones out of the jar and put it back on the shelf. The next day he discovered that the jar again contained some bones. This he took to be a confirmation of his conjecture about a natural phenomenon, so he again fished the bones out and placed the jar, to exclude all possibility of a practical joke, in his wall safe. The result was the same, and he gave the following explanation. When he had cut the echinococcus cysts from the bone, some particles of bone tissue must have gotten into the jar as well. Formalin did not kill their vital properties, which awoke after a lapse of several years and manifested themselves in the growth of bone tissue. He even analyzed the liquid in which this incredible phenomenon had taken place. The article was accompanied by microphotographs of the bones, from which it was obvious that they were not some amorphous mass of bone tissue but a perfectly formed bone with marrow and all the other elements of mature bone, something that takes a long time to form— surely more than a day—and this in a living organism, not some dirty jar.

Imagine a serious scientific journal publishing such absurdities and asking its readers to inform the editors of any similar observations, since they were of great scientific interest. The editor of the journal himself, Studitsky, won notoriety for a sensational experiment. He cut a straight muscle out of an animal's thigh and minced it into a pulp. Then he filled the bed of the muscle with this pulp, and after a while the pulp allegedly formed a functioning muscle of normal structure. For this work, Studitsky and his assistant Alexandra Striganova were awarded the Stalin Prize. Before long, however, Striganova disassociated herself from the work and quarreled with her chief.

The blaze of Lepeshinskaya's triumph was not allowed to wane, and fuel was constantly being added. One day, in summer 1951, I was amazed to see a cavalcade of limousines race past my dacha in the country. Obviously they were bringing some important people. It seemed that this was Lepeshinskaya's eightieth birthday, and Lysenko in person, as well as Zhukov-Verezhnikov and Maisky, director of the Institute of Experimental Biology, and some other bigwigs, had come to congratulate her at her dacha. At a chance meeting some time later, she told me that they had praised her to the skies while she said in reply: "I was not given recognition. I was hampered in my work, and the Virchowians in the Institute of Morphology hounded me out. But I won in the end!" Her words about the Virchowians in the Institute of Morphology sealed the fate of that organization. Soon after the birthday celebrations, the institute was closed.

Years passed. The restoration of the norms of social and political life in the Soviet Union was accompanied by a restoration (though not unopposed) of the norms of true science. It would have been difficult to find a more suitable figure than Lepeshinskaya to discredit Soviet science. This shameful page in our history has been turned, but not forgotten. Still we must not condemn Olga Lepeshinskaya alone. Far more blame should be attached to those careerists and lickspittles among the administrators of science who allowed the free play of her pathological vanity and staged the disgraceful show of her coronation. In this way they made an old and venerable communist, and all of Soviet science as well, the laughing stock of the entire scientific world. Mind you, they have not been punished for it and are still resting on the soft beds they made out of Lepeshinskaya's ridiculous crown of laurels. Meanwhile her "teachings," along with the memory of its author, have been quietly consigned to oblivion.

Moscow, 1975

Index

273

Turgenev, Ivan, 102
Twentieth Party Congress, 67, 150–151, 155, 191, 217
Tyomkin, Yakov, 24
Tyutchev, Fyodor, 18, 222

Ukrainian Academy of Sciences, 239
Unified State Political Directorate (OGPU), 24, 26, 28, 64, 65, 66, 146, 202–203
United States, 10–11, 23, 51, 53, 138, 164, 171, 243, 268, 270
Uspekhi sovremennoi biologii, 271
Utkin, Joseph, 35

Vasilenko, Vladimir, 24, 73, 135, 137–138, 151, 164, 187, 188
Vasilevsky, A. M., 75
Vavilov, Nikolai, 244, 245, 251
Vavilov, Sergei, 245
Velikanov (microbiologist), 64
Vesalius, 227
Vilk, Naum, 82
Vinogradov, Vladimir, 51, 57, 72, 79, 88, 135, 137–138, 151, 164, 200; arrest, 24, 73, 74, 75; vindication, 187, 188; denunciations, 211; as Stalin's doctor, 217–218, 220
Virchowianism, 56, 122, 127, 246, 259, 262, 266, 272
Vishnevsky, Konstantin, 25
Vishnevsky, Yury, 25
Vital substance, theory of, 4, 124, 254–272. *See also* Lepeshinskaya
Vogelson, Lazar, 239
Voice of America, 126
Vovsi, Efim, 162
Vovsi, Miron, 6, 9, 72, 100, 101, 114, 116, 137–138, 142, 144, 161, 164,

173, 239, 269; denunciations, 8, 23, 75, 79, 162, 211; arrest, 73, 74, 143; in prison, 139, 151, 152, 185; vindication, 187, 188; return, 195
Vreden Institute of Traumatology (Leningrad), 82
Vyshinsky, Andrey, 90, 131–132, 218

Wagner, Richard, 36
Weinberg, Severin, 65
Weismanism, 259, 266
Weiss, David, 65
Wilk, Naum, 24
World War II, 121, 162, 172, 220, 225, 240, 244
Writers, campaigns against, 35

Yagoda, H. G., 244
Yakutsk Autonomous Republic, 82
Yegorov, Mikhail, 24, 72, 73, 74, 75, 79, 135, 187, 188
Yeliseev, Professor, 65–66
Young Pioneers, 7, 90, 104, 164
Yukhlov, A., 121, 122, 123

Zakusov, V. V., 187, 188
Zbarsky, Boris, 24, 81, 131, 235
Zdrodovsky, Pavel, 40–41, 65
Zelenin, Vladimir, 24, 81, 89, 135, 164, 187, 188, 203, 239
Zhdanov, A. A., 23, 74, 190, 269
Zhukov-Verezhnikov, Nikolai, 261, 270, 272
Zilber, Lev, 65
Zilov (antisemite), 117, 170, 211, 227–228
Zionism, 49, 79, 172, 211
Zuskin (actor), 67, 68, 244

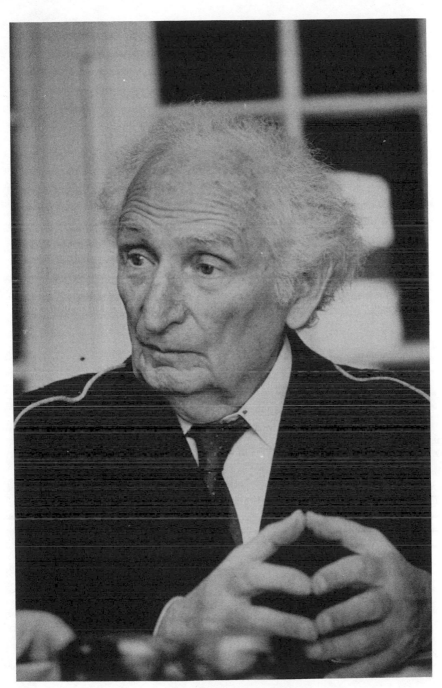

Yakov Rapoport, 1989